RANDOM THOUGHTS WHILE I CAN AND BEFORE I'M GONE

My Al's Story

Dr. Denzel D. Jines, II

TABLE OF CONTENTS

INTRODUCTION

When I started to write down my RANDOM THOUGHTS I wondered who would want to read them. Hopefully anyone feeling depressed will realize there is something everyone is dealing with. Everyone is struggling. A newly diagnosed patient may take away some insight about how attitude helps. Dental and medical students may hopefully see things from a patient's point of reference. My family may see something they've missed. My colleagues may recognize their importance to me and how their friendship and mentorship has been truly appreciated by me. My biker family will recognize the respect I have for our chosen way of life. My LEO family will recognize my gratitude and respect for their sacrifice and courage. I hope my friends see where my foundation in life came from. I am also hoping some reader will find random bits of humor and something to take offense.

The famous quote, "You only live once," has always seemed only partially true to me. My truth as lived daily is, we all die once, unless one is a coward or liar as they die a thousand little deaths daily. The sad truth for many is they never fully live.

The diagnosis of a life-threatening disease or illness should not become the definition of one's life. One's attitude, as expressed in their choice of words and the daily decisions and actions they take, is shaped by life's experiences and one's innate nature. One who is diagnosed with ALS or cancer has a choice to become either a victim or survivor of these illnesses, whether they actually succumb to it or not.

ALS can be a fright-inducing diagnosis, as it comes from an unknown etiology and presents with an unpredictable clinical course. It debilitates its victims, and there are no cures, as of now. Typical life expectancy is two to five years.

I am an ALS patient. My story started long before I was diagnosed with ALS and later cancer. My story has continued long after, and I haven't written the end yet. My story is not sad, nor is it about what ALS has taken from me. My story is about how I live with ALS as a backseat spectator to my life.

I am determined not to be defined by this diagnosis. If anything, I have been defined by my life's work. When asked, "What's up?" I always half-jokingly answer friends by saying, "Fighting disease, stopping crime, and saving lives!"

When I'm asked, "How are you?" my reply is always, "Better than I deserve."

When I was asked, "Why are you still working 'if' you are sick?" Well, there are a whole host of answers to that question. Not jokingly, my first thought is that I still look good. Maybe I'm waiting for something serious. "HELL, I AM JUST TOO DAMN BUSY TO BE SICK!"

I have spent a lifetime growing up in various types of clinics. What I do has not seemed like work in the traditional sense. Yes, I have worked extremely hard at this, but practicing dental medicine is actually the scientific application of art. Just like any artist, I have spent countless hours that require immeasurable personal sacrifices to perfect my art. It is an art not only for a dentist to sculpt dental materials into new tooth structure but to work with the human psyche to endeavor to earn the patients' trust in order to accomplish the artistry. Dental caries (cavities) are holes in teeth created by bacteria (think sugar eating bugs). Dentists are all individuals, and like Picasso or Michelangelo, there are differences in artistic interpretation.

It is an honor and privilege to be entrusted by other people to provide their healthcare as a practicing dental physician (I earned two doctorates, a DMD and an MD). Few jobs come with a title like doctor. It is not just a job or profession; it is what we become.

While practicing in St. Louis, I simultaneously had a second career as a police officer from 1993 until 2016. What little kid doesn't grow up imagining catching the bad guys? I wanted to be a cop way before I wanted to play doctor. Yes, my earliest favorite toy was a Dick Tracy cap gun and shoulder holster by Mattel. I was five. I didn't really think about being a doctor until I was twelve or thirteen. That inspiration just came to me in a dream.

Being a primary healthcare provider is intellectually challenging, emotionally difficult, and physically demanding, though the physical stress isn't from manual labor but the accumulated stress from long hours, sleepless nights, and a sedentary lifestyle. I believe caring for other people is a labor of love, a calling requiring sacrifices that others outside of the field cannot know. Being a doctor is and has been the most consistently rewarding life I know.

Being a police officer requires a similar type of dedication and quick thinking,on your feet, to healthcare. The difference between these two professions may be summed up like this. In medicine if a doctor makes a mistake a patient could potentially die. In Law enforcement if an officer makes a mistake the Officer, the victim and even the bad guy could die. I've never met a law enforcement officer who wakes up looking forward to killing anything, unless it was Deer Season.

Every weekend, I trained with my police departments and worked foot patrol, then traffic, firearms, and defensive tactics trainer, and later drug interdiction with federally assigned DEA officers, and lastly as a Special Deputy with the USMS during fugitive arrest operations. The real rewards for me from police work, besides certainly recognizing First Responders make a positive difference in the lives of our community, are the lifelong relationships and the brotherhood of the alphas.

An example of a "typical" patient contact on a "typical" clinic day could see me removing a large lesion off an elderly man's posterior maxilla due to an infection or abnormal growth in Treatment Room 1, then transitioning to a patient requiring a consult for a lump or bump requiring a biopsy in Treatment Room 2, then off to another patient for a tooth restoration in Treatment Room 3, then rinse and repeat forty to sixty times per day. The one thing that was a welcomed routine after the majority of procedures was that each was followed by a hug and a reminder from the patients that I've been caring for them and their family for over thirty years. Those heartfelt thanks and hugs are more rewarding than what most people will ever receive from any "work." We may all receive paychecks, but mine were literally wrapped in hugs. Unless you are an entertainer and the audience jumps up with applause and adulation, it is difficult for me to think of another type of "work" that so fills the heart. Through my clinic work I received "Chicken Soup for the Soul" daily.

The "typical" contact as an officer with the civilian population was on a different spectrum. Community-based policing is about building positive relationships with the civilian public to reduce criminal activity. In many instances, I served two roles due to my unique background. Being able to offer healthcare advice and let people know they had unknown options garnered trust with civilians. I did see the good in people while working a profession that's called upon to find and deal with the worst of human behavior. Police are routinely expected to go toward the gunfire and to deal with the minute predatory segment of the population that most people would cross the street to avoid. I'm reminded of Paul Harvey's essay on being a cop. Police work was potentially as rewarding as healthcare yet with less, much less, frequency. After a shift, I would oft be reminded of author Dr. Laura Schlesinger's book, *How Could You Do That*. Today's political environment has become toxic to the law enforcement profession. I retired in 2016 when I determined my decreased leg strength could put me—or worst, my partner—at risk in a fight or chase. I was relieved at fifty-eight to close this chapter.

More than missing either profession I have missed the personal interactions with both the public and my professional colleagues, whether they be physicians, dentists, police officers or all the ancillary staff personnel.

I spent my clinic days in the company of wonderful, caring people who I am proud to call friends not just staff and colleagues. I was witness to the promise of the next generation of young millennial doctors through Dr. Cal Harmon and Dr. Michael Czsechin. They provide skilled, high-quality care while demonstrating their tireless work ethic that does great credit to their generation. They have selflessly taken on the responsibility to carry our practice mission well into the future, long after I'm gone.

There are only a few major decisions people will make in their lives. One of the biggest is who we serve with our lives. Once you are outside of yourself, you will easily see why one should stand up in the face of adversity and meet challenges. Serving others has admittedly allowed me to live outside of myself, most of the time.

After my definitive and long-delayed diagnosis with ALS was handed down, I immediately concentrated on the decisions necessary to positively deal with it. It has been my long-held belief that the best way to deal with a threat is to immediately and with ruthless aggression fight it head-on. My first decision was to continue working, which meant continuing to be myself. My only option was, and still is, fighting this.

At first, I had a barely noticeable limp. I would get tested monthly to determine if there was any loss of function or strength. My second decision was, if or when I showed any ALS symptoms or any health crisis, I would stop active hands-on care or active police work. Then, I would seek other avenues of remaining relevant (if only in my head) and remain active in my labors of love. I decided, with the input of my wife and my clinic family and my police chief, that if there was a new way I could participate in patient care or policing, I would do it. If that new way meant mentoring new doctors and students or training officers, I would. I would write down lessons I'd like to pass down to my grandchildren. I would continue to participate in education, as well as the myriad of extracurricular activities I've enjoyed throughout my adult life. In other words, I'd live by the mottos "Carpe diem" and "Live a life that outlives you."

My doctors initiated the (at the time) new IV drug, Radicava. Even though my team of providers was extremely careful, my central port became infected. As a result of that infection, I developed bilateral septic emboli, which are bacterially infected clots, that lodged in both of my lungs. These, in turn, threatened to stop my heart. That night, I took my first ambulance ride as a patient. I later learned from nurses that I was so out of it during the ride that I was, unbeknownst to me, looking at my own EKG and calling out the treatment algorithms for the arrhythmia on the screen. I was admitted to the hospital and treated with IV antibiotics for three weeks.

Right up to that day, I had presented with no functional impediments or clinical deficits; however, I could not nor would I ever risk a patient outcome due to my fragile ego. This was the moment we had planned for, because it is the moral and ethical thing to do. I sadly retired from active patient care in December 2018.

Looking at life through the filter of ALS offers one the opportunity to reevaluate priorities and ideally to focus on making memories living each day to its clichéd fullest. It isn't until you are living it that you realize the cliché is real. It is easy to say, "Hey, we all die!" It is different when the fantasy of a miraculous reprieve is replaced with that new filter of an ALS reality.

I deal with ALS by actively choosing to do whatever, whenever, and however. I adapt to my new realities. While I cannot ignore it, ALS has the backseat on my ride through life. I deal with it by forgiving the past and being grateful for what is left, not what is lost. I am living the best life possible today, right now, and I am eternally better off than I deserve. I am grateful for every second of life still afforded me, here on earth.

CHAPTER 1

FROM SUN TZU'S ART OF WAR—

KNOW THE ENEMY

What is ALS or Lou Gehrig's Disease?
ALS, or Amyotrophic Lateral Sclerosis, also known as Lou Gehrig's Disease, is a nervous system disease that weakens muscles and eventually eliminates voluntary physical function. French neurologist Jean-Martin Charcot discovered the disease in 1869. Since that time, little has changed in the clinical course. It has an average of two to five years of course resulting in death.

There are worse things than death. Everyone reading this will be dead in a hundred years. I would rather live each day as if it is the last thereby, making it the best day instead of worrying about something perfect in the future. Every day is perfect in itself, if lived. Not being able to ride and dive, hold my wife, or hug my kids and grandkids is for me worse than death. I will probably get killed for putting my wife after the dive and ride anyway; or worse, she may want me to go shopping with her. I love to eat GOOD food but ALS eventually steals the ability to eat. I like to talk, and ALS steals that too. I like to breathe, but ALS has a different idea. That's the one that gets you. But before ALS steals your breath away, and not in a good way like the Queen song, this condition steals your smile

1

and ability to join in like you used to. I say "used to" a lot, now, but I also have a lot more that I plan to do.

So, enough of what it does and a little more about what it is. This disease breaks down nerve cells that effect voluntary muscle. Every muscle fiber has its own nerve supply. Once the nerve for any particular muscle fiber is damaged by ALS, there is a loss of that nerve's function that causes the muscle fiber to atrophy. The domino effect is that the nerve dies then the muscle slowly loses its function until it's completely nonfunctional. The cause of this disease whose hallmark is progressive neurodegeneration of nerve cells in the brain and the spinal cord is UNKNOWN.

Amyotrophic Lateral Sclerosis or ALS is a funny-sounding name or word that's all Greek to me. I saw this breakdown of the name in the dictionary that helps one remember the full name instead of just the letters so you can sound like a doctor too. A-myo-trophic comes from the Greek language. The "a" means no, while "myo" means muscle, and "trophic" means nourishment. So, amyotrophic literally means "no muscle nourishment." When a muscle is either unused or starved due to no nourishment, it "atrophies," or wastes away. "Lateral" identifies the areas in a person's spinal cord where portions of the nerve cells that signal and control the muscles are located. As this area degenerates, it leads to scarring or hardening ("sclerosis") in the region. Motor neurons reach from the brain to the spinal cord and from the spinal cord to the muscles.

There are two different types of ALS, sporadic and familial. Sporadic, which is the most common form of the disease in the US, accounts for 90–95 percent of all cases. It may affect anyone, anywhere. Familial ALS (FALS) accounts for 5–10 percent of all cases in the US. Familial ALS means the disease is inherited. This is the type I have, as evidenced by my genetic profile. I have the SOD1 and the MTHFR gene mutations. I am the only known individual in my family to ever-present with a full-blown diagnosis. In families carrying the gene, there is a 50 percent chance each offspring will inherit the gene mutation and may develop the disease. All my doctors performed a good history prior to every physical examination. My history including familial didn't lend itself to a clear diagnosis.

Unfortunately, little has changed in the understanding of what ALS is or how to treat it since Lou Gehrig gave his famous speech in 1939. Recent years have witnessed some new scientific understanding regarding the physiology of this disease; however, its rarity makes urgency take a back seat in funding. Much of the recent research hope has come from the funding brought about by the Ice Bucket Challenge. Since ALS is so rare with a total of 20,000–30,000 cases at any one time in the USA, advancement has been much less than most known disease entities including heart disease, cancer, and HIV/AIDS.

Here are the currently approved meds (2020) along with ALS Association approved resources. There are currently four drugs approved by the US FDA to treat ALS: Riluzole, Nuedexta, Radicava, and Tiglutik. Studies all over the world, many funded by The Association, are ongoing to develop more treatments and a cure for ALS. Scientists have made significant progress in learning more about this disease. In addition, people with ALS may experience a better quality of life in living with the disease by participating in support groups and attending an ALS Association Certified Treatment Center of Excellence or a Recognized Treatment Center. Such Centers provide a national standard of best-practice multidisciplinary care to help manage the symptoms of the disease and assist people living with ALS to maintain as much independence as possible for as long as possible. According to the American Academy of Neurology's Practice Parameter Update, studies have shown that participation in a multidisciplinary ALS clinic may prolong survival and improve quality of life.

To find a Center near you, visit http://www.alsa.org/community/centers-clinics/.

CHAPTER 2

CONVERSATIONS WITH DAD

My personal ALS journey began a couple of weeks before 6 August 1996, while the Summer Olympics were in full swing. I was thirty-eight years old and in private practice in General Dentistry and Oral Medicine. This is a personally important date, because I had been with my first doctor and his assistant, my father and mother, discussing some troubling symptoms, just two weeks prior.

My father and I bonded over Olympic Sports, especially the individual events. There are several Olympic moments that I fondly remember less for the participant's achievements and more for the absolute joy of being in the company of my childhood hero and the pure exuberance we felt together cheering on Jim Hines in the 100m in 1968, or Spitz winning seven golds in 1972, or Dave Waddell coming from behind, or Olga Corbet becoming an Olympic darling, even though she was from the communist USSR, proving sports can transcend politics.

The year 1976 would see not only Bruce Jenner win the Olympic Decathlon but me packing up and heading to college and graduate school before enrolling at Washington University School of Dental Medicine. While a student, I received a commission as an Ensign in the United States Navy. After completion of my naval service and residency training at the University of Virginia, I transitioned to private practice in 1991 and received a commission with the Lebanon Illinois Police Department in 1993. I was living the great American Dream.

My weekends included working on the house; it seemed renovations never ended. Fun activities also included motorcycle riding (a hobby first introduced by family friends in the 1960s), skydiving, SCUBA trips, martial arts training (earned black belt twice), private piloting (including being named the Midwest Search and Rescue K9 Team pilot), and working patrol shifts at the police department (always nights). The boys had added school activities, and we were stretched for time and sleep. It seems I thrived when I was going a 110 percent.

My father was the first Dr. Denzel Jines. I was his first child and the second Dr. Denzel Jines. He was a US Navy veteran and saw combat action in Korea in 1950–53. He graduated from Bradley University and Logan College of Chiropractic Medicine and built the first large multidisciplinary practice in Central Illinois during a time of great prejudice against his chosen field by the established medical community.

He married my mother after WWII and Korea. Their interracial marriage was another fight he chose to take up. We don't always pick who we love; however, the military saw differently, and it put eight years of roadblocks in their way. The Marlon Brando film *Sayonara* was literally their story.

By the time he retired, Chiropractic was gaining acceptance in many hospitals and US service branches, and we were pretty much past the interracial marriage taboos (until recently).

My mother was the original"Tiger Mom". The traditional Japanese discipline and work ethic that she possesses combined with a real spirit of Bushido Code made it necessary for all three of her sons to earn doctorates. There are seven official virtues of

Bushido: courage, righteousness, honesty, benevolence, respect, honor and loyalty. My mother lives them all. Three unofficial virtues piety, wisdom, and care for the elderly characterized her devotion to my father his parents and my uncle. She spent countless hours caring for all of them as their health failed in their final years.

My mother is fearless and her inner personal strength, which comes from unshakable faith, made her a parent of unrivaled discipline who led from the front. She worked along side my father and managed not only his clinic practice but eventually their real estate and investment portfolio. She complemented dads shortfalls and to his credit he knew when to acquiesce to her insight.

Mom wouldn't admit she pressured us more than our father but we all remember her admonitions to never fail in school by getting a "B". When the 1960's counter culture and open drug use started to make news I can remember my mother looking me in the eye and stating," If you ever use drugs or commit crimes you must restore your personal and our whole family's honor and kill yourself." At the time, I thought she meant it.

My father always said he treated the patients that had been failed by the traditional medical community and was happy being that last resort. He eventually owned the buildings that housed several medical practices and the Illinois Dept of Health and the Peoria offices of Blue Cross and Blue Shield. He lectured at the University of Illinois School of Medicine campus in Peoria. He was a Diplomate of the American Board of Chiropractic Orthopedics and certified in Acupuncture. He was doing balloon sinuplasty in the 1970s. His treatments were witnessed by some of my allopathic classmates, and he performed documented "miracles." He could not, nor did he even try to, explain how a blind patient entered his office and left with sight, and another had to be carried in and had been told he would never walk again by his surgeons and literally ran out of my father's clinic after a series of treatments. Witnessing the respect and love he received from patients was the ember that grew within me.

He was one of the first role models who regularly arranged the delivery of food to the needy and showed me the importance of charity. My fondest memories as a young teen are from filling trucks with food around Christmas. His charity made Christmas real. I was told thirty years after the fact by a Peoria police sergeant that my father had provided shoes to him when he was a child delivering papers to my father's office. My father grew up in the depression, where there was great poverty, and he was driven to reach as high on Maslow's hierarchy as possible.

He was a skilled pilot, having earned several ratings beyond instrument flying including flight instructor, commercial, ATP, and multi-engine, to start with. He was a certified diver; however, a ruptured eardrum and cervical fracture shortened his enjoyment of what could have been life-long hobbies. He studied judo and jujitsu in Japan after the war and encouraged my studies in martial arts. As a matter of fact, he was THE role model and yardstick that I measured my own life's work by. I was fortunate to have known who my hero was growing up. He would often say he expected me to do more than he did and give more than he did given. I had it better growing up in post-war affluence. His term was "noblesse oblige." I hope I would have made him proud.

We shared hundreds of clinical talks throughout my early career, as we regularly talked about a plethora of differing clinical issues, and I always cherished his clinical knowledge as well as his business acumen.

The reason I remember this talk was because it was about my own issues, not his. This was the start of my quest for a diagnosis I would never want.

Our talk concerned my own leg muscle weakening. Of course, we thought it was most likely related to lack of sleep, dehydration, electrolyte imbalances, micronutrient deficiency, trace minerals deficiency, and we eventually moved toward musculoskeletal issues or nerve impingement due to scar tissue from injuries (compartmental syndrome) caused by my extracurricular activities. IT WASN'T BECAUSE I ROUTINELY SKIPPED LEG DAY! Maybe the worst case we thought at the time was diabetic neuropathy—after all, he had that—but that was an unlikely diagnosis for me, we both agreed. Neither of us nor my medical physicians would predict ALS.

The second issue we discussed was also related to the weakened legs. I had had a couple of falls in the shower within the weeks leading to our conversation.

There are three ways the body balances, maintaining us erect, and one of the symptoms of ALS in patients is falling. If I closed my eyes in the shower, I would slip. My earliest thoughts on this were related to soap, water, slippery surfaces, even something being organically wrong with my neurological system, like there may be compression on nerves, etc. ALS wasn't a thought yet.

My annual physical examination was scheduled soon after, and I passed. My physicians and I all agreed as everything checked out within normal limits that I'm a healthy male. The symptoms were chalked up to nerve impingement or scar tissue from all the fun I've had, or maybe even a vertebral subluxation, and all I needed was some physical therapy, diet, exercise, massage, chiropractic, and attention to my labs.

Again, ALS wasn't on the radar. Diabetes was on the radar because of family history and because of its deleterious neurological effects, but not ALS. My father would say, "Common things happen commonly." In other words, a diagnosis of ALS, a rare disease that doesn't fit my particular clinical presentation, would be what we call a zebra diagnosis.

During our conversations, we also discussed his altered gait, which manifested years before, and his lower extremity wasting, which at the time was determined to be a result of Type II Diabetes.

Obviously, his health issues were a priority, since I appeared to be the picture of health. We routinely discussed how he was failing, with several of the devastating health issues related to diabetes. He passed away from a stroke on 6 August 1996.

In retrospect, my legs now look like his legs. He occasionally choked on food, and his arms, which had been muscular (he routinely beat all a Trophied as well my high school football friends in arm wrestling and curls).

It was easy to brush off his wasting to his diabetes, which he didn't control, and his choking to eating and talking too much.

I miss our conversations.

CHAPTER 3

DECADES CHASING A SHADOW—ALS

After my father passed, I cranked up the intensity of my routine. I already worked out with moderate intensity throughout my adult life. My wife and I mostly ate organic, with a careful, plant-based diet. I rode my bike, ran, lifted, benched over 300lbs, and I didn't skip leg days. I trained with my friends on the police department's Emergency Response Team (SWAT), which included not only firearms, martial arts, emergency medicine, and defensive tactics, but also HazMat and disaster training. Well into my fifties, there were no overt signs that I just was not functionally right except for a slight limp. I have several friends who have had lifetime chronic injuries similar to mine, so our old "war wounds" and their resulting scars and arthritis and limping were just considered par for the course.

My muscles of facial expression would occasionally quiver, and my leg muscles would ripple in waves. My medical training would describe this as a form of neuropathy, but the frequency and duration of these symptoms had remained the same since I was in my early twenties. My friends at the gym would remark that my body twitches were visually like a racehorse twitching. The muscles around my eyes, eyebrows, and eyelids would wiggle visibly and looked occasionally like I was winking to the beat of the music, and this was all involuntary. Maybe too much caffeine! Nope, I will never give it up. I drink black coffee and have since I was a 3-year-old hyperkinetic kid. Coffee was a safer treatment for hyperkinetic (today's ADD) kids. ALS is so rare, it still wasn't even in the differential.

I was much more concerned about the leading cause of death in the USA, which was and still is heart disease. I worked to prevent heart disease following a plant-based diet recommended by Pritikin, Ornish, Mirkin, Greger, all medical physicians at the forefront of preventive medicine. The best part about preventive medicine is that following the dietary guidelines outlined by the above-named medical researchers prevents obesity, diabetes, heart disease, and even hypertension, which in turn decreases the likelihood of kidney diseases, strokes, and heart attacks.

The fitness craze of the past three decades has brought with it a great deal of growth in our knowledge of human performance. We now know that 70 percent of healthcare dollars are spent on illnesses brought on and exacerbated by lifestyle. That is why I never believed the narrative that the USA has a healthcare crisis. The USA has a self-induced health crisis.

While obesity levels have actually risen, social pressure has pushed for anti-bullying and body acceptance of the curves associated with being overweight to outright obese. The sicker the population has become, the wider the "normal" ranges in lab values have become.

ALS has been shown to affect military members with twice the frequency of the general public. It is also seen in extreme athletes with a higher rate than non-athletes. I spent three years on an aircraft carrier and trained hard to avoid heart disease. ALS was never on the radar.

Part of my private practice was to tie in the systemic effects of oral diseases upon the entire body. I therefore practiced what

I was preaching and wanted to be an example of health to my smoky, friends, and patients. No one likes taking diet and lifestyle advice from a 300lbs smoking doctor, which begs the questions, "Self-aware much? Double standards much? Hypocrisy much? Do as I say, not as I do much?!"

In 1994, I ran a relay with two of my police department friends Joe and Keith as part of a shooting competition. Upon completion of my leg, there were people who said, "You ran so fast! I had no fricking idea!"I was thinking I was a sprinter in high school and ran with my college team until the choice became crystal clear to either try to make the track team—knowing I would never be world class fast—or focus on academics. I chose academics. I did take the lessons learned from competition and training to know my body. In 1994, I was fast—not Olympic fast, but if you ran from me during an arrest, I would usually surprise everyone and catch you. By the way, back in the day, when somebody ran, not only did you get arrested, but you got arrested tired and sweaty.

In 2000, I ran 3 minutes below the state qualifying times required for new police academy recruits. Regardless of the timed results, I had trouble with my stride and thought it must be the shoes or the track pants were too tight. I was thrilled that my performance was strong. That same year, I ran a race against my sons in front of the house. The younger teens, fifteen and sixteen, were challenging the old man, and I was going to teach them a lesson. I had foot drop throughout our 100-yard race, and almost fell twice. I also couldn't put my stride into second gear. Again, I assumed it must be my sweatpants or shoes. My sons destroyed me by about ten yards. ALS was just a Gary Cooper movie subject.

I looked, at forty-two years old, like any forty-year-old, except maybe younger and stronger. My waist was still 31–32 inches, and chest was 48. My bench was 300, and my biceps were 18 inches. Nothing wrong with me is what my annual physical would show. What the exam failed to show was the pride in my sons or the hurt ego that comes from knowing I'm getting older. Again, no news was good news, as whatever it is, it's not looking serious or anything like ALS. It's the shoes. I could get them the next time. Just wait. Ego is such a fragile entity, anyway. I should be proud of them, and I was.

The year 2008 saw the loss of my youngest son Eric. Many lose their lives in direct service to this nation. Eric's sad death occurred after he returned; however, his life was lost years before, during his time in Iraq. As a young boy, he stated he wanted to grow up and be a Marine or SEAL. He was the youngster everyone knew would be a superstar. He was an Honor Student and a gifted musician who was inducted into the Who's Who of American High School Students. He was Mike Utechtt's first Kajukenbo Blackbelt and trained for MMA. He was someone who loved learning. He was "that kid" who asked a million questions. Joe C. Paulfrey, my best man and police partner, had him ready for the USMC when it came to small arms. When his DI asked who, what, and where did he get all his prior training, as it pertained to tactical firearms use, he told them Joe and my dad. His DI shook my hand at his boot camp graduation ceremony. Eric excelled at everything he did. His spirit was exceptional enough that he was chosen as one of the students to meet Pope John Paul on his STL visit. As a musician, his band made waves and gained recognition but 9/11 happened, when some people did something(Islamic terrorists flew hijacked commercial flights and destroyed the World Trade Center and the Pentagon), and the patriotic fervor along with teen angst brought his enlistment to fruition. He left for Iraq in 2004–5 and returned here 75 percent disabled. The VA unknowingly administered the coup de grâce by iatrogenic means, providing him prescriptions for drugs like Paxil, Seroquel, Prozac, and Clonipin simultaneously. Any medically trained friends know this is contraindicated. Gone was the light-hearted, bright-eyed, caring, and loving embodiment of the All American Youth, and born was the drug-addled zombie that was neither alive nor dead. His sacrifice cost not only his life offered up to the mantel of freedom but his family's sanctity as well. Mary's older brother and protector, Denzel's younger brother and best friend, had taxed his entire personal world through his devolution. His passing caused a rift that tore apart lives and changed the course of our collective futures. Not a day goes by that we don't miss him.

The next several years were the most emotionally and physically stressful in my life. The progression of my leg weakness was steady; however, I treated it as just the march of time. Anyway, all testing always showed I was strong.

I remained nose to the grindstone, seeing patients four days a week with students just one semester per year and working weekends with the police department and training.

In 2010, a photographer said I should capture my physique, since it wasn't usual for men my age, and at that age, it may go fast, he jokingly pressured. I agreed to his request as I also wanted to capture a snapshot of time (vanity) and possibly use it as an inspiration to patients and friends, like many of my favorite bodybuilding role models.

During this session, I noticed my calf muscles would not flex as they were usually so well defined that I had actually received unsolicited compliments from strangers, including professional athletes. That day, they just would not do what was commanded. I had replaced lifting on leg days to running so I thought that was what caused it. So, yes, I skipped leg day occasionally, but this was dramatic. I was never able to repeat my previous lifts, and my range of motion decreased as far as squat depth, and even raising on my toes, until eventually, I couldn't do a toe raise at all.

All of this led to more exams, where all function tests done clinically were normal, and I was actually testing above normal in strength. Every exam would exceed test parameters, so the doctors, including neurologists, concluded I was okay. There seemed to be just some unknown deficit, but there was nothing to worry about.

In 2012, while diving, I had an equipment malfunction that caused me to go from 130ft depth during a wreck dive to the surface in a few seconds. Luckily, I hadn't been at depth for more than a few seconds before a valve in my buoyancy compensator devise (BCD) malfunctioned, causing instant inflation of my BCD and an immediate decrease in depth surfacing like a submarine breaching. This would later happen a second time, not to me but to my wife, Darla, while at 80ft looking at a 500lbs grouper and huge school of fish off the Florida coast. Luckily for her, there were no ill side effects.

In my case, I suffered a debilitating "thunderclap" headache a few hours later. I thought my head was going to explode. It was serious enough that I had to schedule an appointment with Barnes Neurologists as soon as I got home. *Had I had a stroke?* I wondered, *or delayed nitrogen sickness?* While extremely unlikely, my mind still was on overdrive because of the severity and sudden onset of pain. I had taken precautions and, luckily, that was the only incidence of a headache, especially like that. ALL tests returned NORMAL. I mentioned the other neurological symptoms, but just like all previous evaluations, they returned normal. I was normal? No news is always good news.

I kept pressing, and again, the diagnosis was something musculoskeletal, and PT was recommended. I also did chiropractic this time with Dr. Mathew Worth, who is also a neurology specialist in his field.

His EMG tests showed abnormalities, and he referred me back to Barnes, where the same tests revealed the same results. So, within a period of weeks, I had gone from "nothing to worry about" to "there's something wrong." I was now diagnosed with MMN multifocal motor neuropathy and prescribed IVIG.

After one treatment, I regained strength in my toes. I used to be able to pick up a dime with my toes. Again, for the first time in years, I could do it again. I was able to move them with purpose.

The diagnosis came without notice and in the most round-about ways. My insurance refused to continue treatment with IVIG until I was reevaluated. My neurologist at Barnes redid the previous testing and changed my diagnosis to ALS. Just like that, there was no more treatment that I believed had a positive effect. I was given the standard talk on ALS, including a talk about getting my affairs in order and the two to five years of timeline.

I tried to pay for the IVIG myself but was turned down. I then went to another medical school SLU, where the local ALS Association is located, for confirmatory diagnosis, and went through the evaluation and testing process again and received the same results. ALS. This was June 2015.

My wife was in the clinic when my neurologist at the time said, "You must accept this diagnosis and prepare for the inevitable, which may be death within a short time."

To date, there is nothing that actually treats and cures this illness. The prognosis has not changed since it was described and named after baseball legend Lou Gehrig.

I was offered the new wonder drug, Radicava, that came to market after the Ice Bucket Challenge. Its side effects are altered gait (I already had that) and dysphagia (swallowing difficulty, which I didn't have).

I used it until my port became infected and my insurance company refused to cover the $150,000/year cost. The insurance company's rationale was that I don't need it, as described earlier.

ALS Ice Bucket Challenge Founder Peter Frates passed away recently. This is sad news indeed. Peter battled this as best he could. His contribution is the epitome of taking the fight forward. His was an example of living positively despite adversity.

Peter Frates started the Ice Bucket Challenge in 2014. From his efforts, a newer medication Radicava was brought forth. It may slow the illness. Unfortunately, no one knows if it will last more than a short time.

Peace out.

CHAPTER 4

CARPE DIEM, MEMENTO MORI

I have oft wondered why patients, when given a particular diagnosis, react one of two particular ways. I don't mean in the immediate seconds upon hearing a diagnosis like ALS or Alzheimer's or Cancer, but in a particular way, a patient then processes the information and goes about either living/fighting or dying with it as a result.

I have lived by a motto immortalized by Robin Williams in his film *Dead Poets Society*, Carpe Diem . . . Seize the Day. Though it was put into a singular expression in the film, my daily activities and lifestyle were already an expression of this concept. Another way I personally expressed this idea was in body art. I have the expression "CARPE DIEM and MEMENTO MORI and LIVE A LIFE THAT OUTLIVES YOU, What's your excuse?" inked on me, as well as my entire life's story. So far.

How does a diagnosis of a serious health issue and Carpe Diem relate? This should be quite obvious. From all the preceding storyline, I hope one comes away with the idea that they have a choice. Anger and happiness are by choice. One chooses to seize the moment and steer toward calmer seas, or one chooses to succumb to any threat by giving in.

Success in improving one's quality of life requires owning the temple they live in.

The individuals I have seen that handle illness well are the same ones that handle life well in general. They are for the most part (prior to diagnosis) active, happy people with faith (note that I didn't write religious) who were previously proactive in their own health or who become their own best healthcare advocates by engaging with me and their other doctors to take their own health seriously.

My patients that are survivors seldom just do whatever their doctors tell them without studying exactly what's happening, especially in the days of Google and WebMD. My survivors are not defined by their illnesses but live high quality, inspired, productive lives in spite of them. Yes, they may be more preoccupied with their conditions as they alter their lifestyles to accommodate for the disabilities thrust upon them, but my survivor patients continually embrace the life they lived prior to their diagnoses and continue to plan for future adventures instead of a life of acquiescence to diminished quality of life. They seize the day and live life to its fullest, whether it is climbing that mountain, or checking off an item on their Bucket List, or getting up and marching off to work. This latter group, those that continue to work, are usually the luckiest ones in that they that love their work or are those defined by it— doctors, artists, writers—those who are lucky enough to actually labor at the thing they love.

I've personally known ALS patients and cancer survivors who expressed a positivity in actions and words that allowed them to face the worst without fear nor complaint.

My patients who weather the storms poorly instead of dancing in the rain usually tell me to do whatever I think best as they possess no desire to be involved in the decision-making process. These patients usually look for a magic pill to cure their ills (most medicines cover up symptoms of disease rather than cure it) so they can continue their own self-abusive, unhealthy lifestyle. They offer up a myriad of excuses with a plethora of rationalizations for why they cannot make the hard choices regarding owning the machine they live in. I often ask patients, "Where exactly are you planning on residing after you wear this particular body out?" These patients routinely allow the abundance of their hearts to leak out of their mouths. They say things that belie their disdain for their work, relationships, and material possessions. They are not thankful, nor grateful or forgiving in nature. They do not Carpe Diem. I know that hurts a few feelings, but the only person who can change your outlook is in your mirror.

Whenever I have given a patient bad news, I have always presented it as an opportunity to make choices and sometimes changes. When I say you can do something and they say they just cannot or are not willing to make any changes, it reminds me of the dozens of times I have looked into their eyes and said, "Your prognosis really depends on which one of us is going to be your doctor."

So, what type of patient are we to become? For me, today, as long as it's not illegal, immoral, or fattening, I guess I'll just *carpe diem quam minimum credula postero.*

This is yet another saying I've had inked, along with another that is the WHY.

CARPE DIEM because MEMENTO MORI.

"Seize the day because you may be dead tomorrow."

CHAPTER 5

SO I HAVE ALS, WHAT'S NEXT

ALS does not define me even though it may kill me I have a choice on how I live with it.

Wow, I get great parking, now! When I go to Disney, they are extra nice. Deep down, a voice told me, "I should have done this years ago." I haven't changed since that day. ALS has changed a few things but not me.

The workouts had to be reduced in order to not injure muscles that will no longer get bigger and stronger but instead will atrophy. I still worked out, but the goals are different. I'm trying to maintain functional strength and not build my body. My new focus was to never induce soreness the next day. Soreness means I overdid it, so tomorrow I'll be weaker instead of stronger.

I chose to just keep going the way I always have. I was enjoying life, so why change? I will most certainly adapt to what is occurring, just like in a fight, where one's tactics change to fit the terrain or the opponent or any other surprises that are thrown in. Except for the great parking. I want great parking.

I was performing dental and oral surgical procedures, consulting with several referring dental and medical clinics daily, and was at my clinical prime when this diagnosis was given. Our decision was that I would remain in practice as long as I showed no deficit in function other than the slight limp. I received the new drug, Radicava, and developed a port infection, as well as decreased leg function. I stopped the treatment and stopped seeing patients four years after my original diagnosis. The insurance experts next said they would not cover ALS meds because they determined I did not have ALS. I'm cured! Well, my clinical experts, who have evaluated, tested, scored, imaged, shocked, biopsied, and otherwise put me through a more rigorous diagnostic regimen, from both major clinical centers in St. Louis, the VA, and The Missouri Brain and Spine Institute, say different.

I've maintained my license, and I continue doing continuing education and write for *Dental Clinical Pearls* website. However, I will no longer enjoy the personal, intimate interaction that comes from the honor and trust of treating a patient.

One door closes and others open. I believe in Churchill's admonition, "Never quit." We all die, but many never fully live, so my goal has been to "live a life that outlives me." Another saying I mentioned earlier that I have Vitamin Inked onto my canvas.

I retired from the police department when I could no longer aid my partners on the street. The year 2016 saw my last shift. I could still roll on the mat and continue to do so, but I walked with a more noticeable limp that gives the impression that I am weak to the predatory criminals we occasionally interacted with. My partners continued to invite me to ride along, saying it's not the running but the common sense of community-based policing that makes it okay to still report for duty. Common sense is 99.99 percent of the job, with the mundane being the rule of the day. It is just that 0.01 percent of the time where sheer adrenaline-fueled chaos interjects itself, and that could occur anytime. It was that 0.01 percent that made me stop for the same reasons I stopped seeing patients. I would never be able to forgive myself if my fellow officers needed me, and I was not there.

I have remained active in several other activities, like the afore-mentioned writing for *Dental Clinical Pearls*, guiding my clinical staff toward new accreditations in sleep medicine, firearms train-ing of police, and my motorcycle club, where I was elected presi-dent of the Southern Illinois chapter or the Reguladores LEMC in 2019. My only acquiescence to ALS, in regard to riding, has been the transition from two wheels to three.

Four wheels move the body, but two wheels move the soul. Three wheels are a great compromise, as I get many of the ben-efits of four wheels like increased stability, yet I'm still getting wind therapy. I have always said you never see motorcycles parked in front of psychiatrist's offices.

The daily mantra when I wake up goes something like this:

ALS does not define me. It may kill me, but until then, I'm me. I will choose to live my best life on my own terms!

On any given day after I was forced to retire from active prac-tice, my life devolved from a rigorously scheduled affair of treat-ing patients, teaching students, answering calls, family duties, and police work to writing clinical and political posts and traveling with my motorcycle club to home renovation to infinity and beyond!

Living life with ALS is not a one-dimensional struggle. ALS does not eliminate the requirement to meet one's obligations, whether they be matrimonial, financial, or spiritual, nor does it kill the desire I have to enjoy each day, because today is the best day and best time to live.

I also discovered not only the great parking benefits, but I was also now qualified for other benefits that I had never expected to receive, even though I have been employed either part-time or full-time for forty-six years.

ALS is an automatic Social Security Disability and Medicare approval as well as Veterans Affairs 100 percent disability rating that is service related!

CHAPTER 6

THE BIRTH OF RANDOM THOUGHTS

The remainder of this story will be my Random Thoughts on various topics while living life since my diagnosis. Regardless of ALS, I am still dealing with important stuff like family, dentistry, medicine, law enforcement in the USA, motorcycles, and politics. Every day offers a cornucopia of new opportunities of such diverse spheres as to lend credence for the concept of the random nature of the universe, and ergo, Random Thoughts.

By the way, just because I am an ALS patient doesn't mean I am not interested in life and politics outside of this disease. Right now, it would seem Plato was right. Too many have ignored political involvement, thereby ensuring we are being ruled over by inferior intellects. My advice is "Read a book and wake up."

Doctor means teacher. Any writing I have done throughout my career has been to teach. To that end, I have attempted to make every point within this storyline one that allows the reader an opportunity to garner information that they may use.

Random Thought: I was asked, "Hey! You seem to be doing well. What is your regimen?"
Before and after my diagnosis, I worked out with a combination of cardio, weights, and martial arts. My cardio training consisted

of walking, elliptical and treadmills, and circuit training lifting. Off days, I'd do core training utilizing a wonder wheel ab roller, planks, and heavy bag. This regimen was my staple from 1979 until now.

After my diagnosis, I was determined to work out with even more intensity but there was an issue. With ALS, there is an increase in oxidative stress on nerve cells, and working out increases oxidative stress. ALS patients exhibit decreased levels of all their naturally occurring antioxidants. Therefore, ALS patients don't recover and get stronger after workouts. They can actually get weaker. As nerve tissue is damaged, muscle cells and fibers atrophy. Think: nerve dies, then muscle dies. If you don't work out, you atrophy too. That's the rub. I had to change workouts drastically.

The current literature suggests light workouts that don't go to failure are the best middle ground and help maintain function. If you are sore the next day, you did too much!

I also supplement with IV Meyers cocktail, IV glutathione, IM sermorelin growth hormone replacement peptides 2,6, and IM testosterone.

I am also taking oral supplements using liposomal glutathione, turmeric, collagen, B vitamins, JuicePlus, coQ 10, CBD, and other prescribed nutritional supplements.

I'm not taking any prescription ALS medication. I tried Radicava. All my current issues in weakness and altered gait accelerated immediately after starting Radicava. I was progressing slowly and didn't start this medication until rather late into my diagnosis, approximately two years in. I was still climbing stairs prior to starting it. I stopped this medication and will wait for something else. It may help different cases but didn't help me, and that's my opinion. In the meantime, I'll continue walking as much as possible, working out, eating well, and doing all the nutrition therapy along with treatments from my chiropractic neurologist, as well as my ALS medical team.

My goal is to make everything within my control better, healthier and stronger.

We all die. I just don't want it to be my fault!

I'm not advocating any specific therapy, nor recommending any supplement. I am recommending we all become our own best health advocate. Adopting a healthy lifestyle can only help. There is no downside to a healthy lifestyle.

CHAPTER 7

RANDOM THOUGHTS—LIFE GOES ON

I was asked by a well-intentioned young man, "If you got a disease that makes you weak, why not hit the weights?"

While this question alludes to the previous chapter, not everyone approaches ALS from the same reference point.

Have you ever noticed the next generation believes everything started from the day they were born? The next younger generation invented cool and has the best music, sex, fashion, whatever. Whatever!

How many times have I used an example that the unfortunate audience possessed no reference point for? Recent examples include . . . who is John Wayne, Steve McQueen, Dean Martin, Chuck Yeager, Washington, Adams, Jefferson, Monroe, Paine, Henry, The Godfather, John, Paul, George, Ringo, John, Paul, Mark, even Judas?

Everyone has a struggle or challenge in life: mentally, spiritually, physically, financially. EVERYONE.

When we lack reference and perspective to one another's struggles, we may, unfortunately, ignore, overlook, or remain indifferent to them. Having compassion for one another and being empathetic are not always the first reactions because many lack a reference point to another's struggles.

Hopefully, this won't be the case to those that read my Random Thoughts today on ALS.

ALS, or Lou Gehrig's Disease, is a degenerative nerve disease that usually ends in death within two to five years of diagnosis. It kills the nerves that are responsible for all voluntary movements like communication, expression, and breathing. The patient remains fully cognizant of every word uttered, every sound heard, everyone and everything seen, but is left unable to say, "I hear that, I see that, or I love you." The patient diagnosed with ALS may eventually be trapped inside a body, all the while fully aware of what goes on around him or herself without the ability to interact.

The clinical course can be extremely rapid, and in a few rare cases like Stephen Hawking, the progression is very slow. Professor Hawking led a full life, giving hope to others with this condition that they too can remain productive through the gifts that spring forth from their minds in the remaining time they have.

The trick is to not give up hope, nor to become defined as ALS.

ALS constantly reminds those afflicted of what they are losing. Great NFL players, who are unquestionably superhuman, can win a Super Bowl and then mere months later be unable to walk, talk, or breathe when afflicted with ALS. They are reminded daily of their fragility, like any other ALS patient. This is the moment I've been describing throughout this book. Dwelling on what is lost is spirit and soul-crushing. Learning to be truly grateful for what is left is a gift.

For me personally, this has been a mental, scientific, and spiritual battle with the most frustrating enemy I have ever faced—or a very close second, when compared to losing a child, or third when asking for that first kiss, or fourth, or fifth or . . . Yes, it's tough, but it is not defining.

Daily, I look and recognize I can no longer do XYZ . . . However, even if I can no longer perform surgery, as my wife says, "You ARE still a doctor. You ARE still a father. You ARE still MY husband. You ARE still all those things to me."

She is correct. When dealing with ALS or Cancer or Cystic Fibrosis or any human frailty, don't let "it" define who you are.

Remain involved. Be for the next generation a conduit of information, knowledge, and hopefully wisdom, so they have a reference point beyond the tip of their own noses.

CHAPTER 8

RANDOM THOUGHT—ALS AND FAITH

Nothing like a health crisis or a mugger with a gun to introduce one to faith. I'm not talking religion or paperback self-help new age spiritualism. I'm talking faith.

The cool kids today say they are atheists or agnostics. Okay, whatever makes you feel smart. I choose to have faith. I choose to believe there is more that we cannot see. One thing I have learned throughout my life is I that don't know everything, and I know I don't know everything.

I don't really think we are all alone. This is a personal choice that's biblical. It is a choice I made that is comforting. We are all individuals who go through our daily lives with individual struggles and challenges and eventually must come to terms with things like mortality. It is at this juncture that we each go through that moment: that passing through the veil, that stepping to the other side, you know, we croak or—more delicately put—we assume room temperature, and it's an individual's alone moment. Even if it is on a doomed flight, we all go individually.

It is comforting to believe we are not alone and that there is a constant companion with us throughout our lives. God. With that notion, I think we can make sense of things easier. It is between you and God. Now, what each individual decides to make of God is the beauty and the agony of human freedom. Our Free Will allows us to believe God is a guy on a cloud with a beard pulling on puppet strings, or just sitting on a throne watching and waiting to judge, or maybe a benevolent or malevolent being ready to bestow untold wealth or eternal damnation upon our heads. Some believe God is a form of alien intelligence or a spirit of limitless knowledge and supernatural power. Well, we can even believe we know God personally and have a relationship, like a loving involved parent, or like the parents that ignore their children, and vice versa.

Wouldn't it be nice to just know and understand we don't know what we don't know, so instead of judging and condemning everyone else's knowledge and relationships of their God, we would learn to actually live the golden rule?

We are given the freedom to choose to believe, and it is an individual choice. Whether there is or isn't a God is an individual's choice they each must make.

I would rather live a life hopeful there is a God instead of one without, only to learn later, oops, there really is. That's why I choose to believe there is a heaven and hell, and that there's a judgment that happens later. Knowing that my father would whip my butt for doing something stupid like committing a crime or destroying my own life with drugs etc., helped shape me into an individual who respects the rule of law and is willing to sacrifice and work for a better future for his grandkids.

Without the concepts of a living God, it is easy to see human nature take hold and savagery takes reign through lawless brutality.

It seems the two sides of this debate are lining up to determine where human civilization ends up. Rational thought is being replaced by emotional groupthink and denial of reality by political officeholders. An apathetic public more interested in sports has not paid attention to the unique nature of the Founding of the USA and its history. They have allowed a country whose motto is "In God we trust" to be separated from the only source of our rights, willing to trade those very rights for temporary security offered by man (government). They have given the responsibility of the exercise of those rights away, enabling their own children to be indoctrinated into denying God, hating our nation, and electing officials who not only possess inferior intellects themselves but who actively deny the benevolence of God and invite every suicidal evil known yet to man.

To me, or should I say for me, faith allows us to see beyond physical limits. I have seen medical miracles that doctors from the various hospitals I have worked and even taught in cannot explain: cancers disappearing without medical intervention, and blind persons regaining their sight with no medical explanation.

I know centering oneself spiritually can have positive measurable effects on overall health, but I personally have found the Bible to be a useful How-To Manual or Instruction Guide. I have said it quite often that ALS does not define me; however, I do feel its effects. I could easily let the daily falls or the painful cramps that indicate more muscle death or the choking (the scariest symptom) really get to me. I could let the image in the mirror where once I saw eighteen-inch arms and legs so muscular a few pro athletes would compliment me and where I now see deteriorating flesh really get to me. I could let ALS steal the joy Darla Porter-Jines and I had on the beach by comparing it to the last time we were on the beach and I went a little farther than this time. I could let the images and negative voice (ALS steals relentlessly) gain a solid foothold on my psyche and become disillusioned so as to not try again later.

Everyone who is in my inner sanctum of friends knows I have dieted and exercised my entire adult life, but that is not enough. With ALS, there is nothing from the physical aspect that I have not done. This is the exact point where faith (notice I didn't say religion) can make a difference. Every page of the Bible stresses winning. We say sin, the Bible says salvation. We say sickness, the Bible says through Him we can find healing. We say death, and through the Bible, we can learn there is everlasting life. My favorite time of the year and the favorite holiday is upon us. I pray everyone who reads this finds a way to find Peace and Joy.

Faith helps take the burden away, especially with health issues like ALS.

CHAPTER 9

RANDOM THOUGHT—RELATIONSHIPS AND

SECOND CHANCES

My review of literature reinforces a simple truth as it relates to ALS and team approach care. It is essential for an improved quality of life. What is most essential is the daily and hourly interaction of family and friends.

After the death of a child, many marriages undergo so much turmoil that they fail. I won't blame the failure of my first marriage on my son. I may as well blame it on my eldest son or, hey, how about my daughter?

My two other children don't deserve that. Both are now successful adults. Denzel III is a supervisor at the US Navy Recruit Training Base at Great Lakes. He is a decorated US Army combat Veteran who returned from Iraq and graduated with Honors from my alma mater Southern Illinois University, Edwardsville. He next studied for his MBA in Chicago. He is married to the beautiful Sophia and they have three great kids, Addyson, Bristol, and Denzel IV.

Our daughter Mary was born on my fortieth birthday. She too is an honor student, making National Honor Society, Illinois

State Scholar, National Merit Scholar, and currently finishing with Honors at St. Louis University, and we are waiting to see if she will be living abroad next year as a Fulbright Scholar.

Relationships after divorce have been written about and described in detail, yet all relationships are a unique story of individuals interacting, learning, growing, moving on or moving in . . . you get it. Each relationship can run the entire gambit of human interaction.

Relationships, including marriages, end for a whole variety of reasons, and it's up to each of us to pick up the pieces of a shattered life, hopefully, learn from our experiences, and move forward with our lives. I am thankful for the thirty years I was married, as there are, in retrospect, more positive blessings than negative moments. We are in mutual agreement on our grown children, we work together to help them, and we have put the acrimony and bitterness aside and replaced it with respect and prayers for each other. We both grew and are happy now in our respective lives. Being friendly and finding the ability to be cordial not only brings peace, but it is the only choice we desired mutually to take.

I recently gave her (my ex) my blessings as she remarried a guy she, my daughter, and Adele described as exactly like me—know it all (but in a good way) retired USAF flight instructor Full Bird (military lingo), exactly the kind of guy I am.

I was blessed as well, to have found a girl who spoke to my heart, reintroduced me to God and all the possibilities of faith, reminded me of that perfect love that forgives and was always alive in me, had I only opened my eyes. Darla has given me strength and confidence to again face all the challenges life brings as I truly know I am never alone. My relationship with myself has improved, as we both seek guidance from outside ourselves and place trust where it should rightfully be.

Everyone, absolutely everyone, has personal struggles, conflict, and battles they face that most of the rest of the world will never see. We usually treat the world as if everyone else is doing better and we are the only ones struggling. It is easy to allow negative thoughts to be our inner dialogue, and we often talk ourselves out of success.

Darla has been my blessing and champion, always giving me a pep talk, always the right word of encouragement, always that approving look and supportive touch. Because of Darla, I believe in second chances and in a bright future that awaits. Because of her tireless unconditional devotion, I am ready to start living again, right now, every second of every day, honoring God, my family, and especially her. She is the rock and foundation of my world. I have been blessed to have her enter my life and complement me. She truly completes me.

We dated before my diagnosis with ALS and married over two years after being diagnosed.

CHAPTER 10

RANDOM THOUGHTS—DOCTORS, HIPSTERS,

AND INK

ALS wreaks havoc upon the body's function and appearance. I had spent my entire adult life practicing a healthy lifestyle. A side benefit of working out was and is that you look good naked. I worked out not only to be healthy, but I also did it to sculpt a certain physical appearance.

As ALS has stolen my body, I have chosen to use ink as a way of changing my body's appearance on my terms.

I retired in 2016 after over twenty-six years in Law Enforcement, which was the first love even if not my primary profession. I also worked full-time as a dentist and physician and was a former clinical instructor of Plastic Surgery at St. Louis U. I wrote this about INK and wanted to share it here with my LE and healthcare families.

Random Thoughts on Hipsters Getting Tattoos and Those Whose Ancestors Have Used Ink for Centuries

I was asked by a resident physician about my ink. He clandestinely offered he has one, and he'd like to get more but was afraid of the stigma that comes from a generation that grew up being taught the only people with tattoos are veterans and convicts. I told him about older medical texts stating just that.

I am torn emotionally when it comes to younger people with limited life experiences permanently celebrating a spring-break fling by putting someone's name where everyone can see it, especially if it is cheap ink and the match made in heaven is over in forty-eight hours.

I explained that I waited a lifetime and built my practice and career, teaching the next generation of young providers and playing by the old rules. I have always, since my early twenties, planned to illustrate my life's story, accomplishments, and family, like my Japanese Samurai ancestors who were the Last Samurai of the 1870s. I have seen colorized pictures of their entire bodies covered in traditional ink. Now, in my sixties and bearing witness to the effects of ALS and cancer on one's physique, I use my opportunities to illustrate my story as a means to maintain my control on how my body changes

I do believe recent polls that show the general public does not hold a negative view of doctors and police and military veterans and nurses and people who have tattoos. I do believe as well that had I started early, my ink would have had a negative effect on my career. I felt the sting of prejudice regarding my race and clothing choices in my early days of practice. During my residency at the University of Virginia, while I was serving as the Chief Resident, I had an African-American female upon introduction respectfully ask for a "White" doctor. This was upon introduction, let alone treatment. She took one look at this dark-skinned doctor and before I could speak, I just said, "Please take no offense, but I want a white doc."

Today, this type of prejudice is almost completely gone, and as society has progressed and as the younger generation gets inked earlier (names of that fling can be covered or erased), hopefully with plenty of thought, you will see industry leaders and the leaders of most fields sporting visible tattoos.

The story and illustrations continue with Greg J Schaefer and Jeremy Lambert doing all the work.

CHAPTER 11

RANDOM THOUGHTS—ALS RIDES A

MOTORCYCLE

Reguladores LEMC: A History of a Great American Law Enforcement Motorcycle Club

This club got its own chapter because it is deserved.

Riding is quintessentially a pure expression of traditional American Heritage and All American Freedom. Riding with a group of individuals who share a common passion for motorcycling along with a shared profession such as First Responders and Military Veterans gives that expression of freedom a deeper personal meaning. Approximately 1 percent of the population serves in the military, signing a contract that should the time come, they may in fact pay the ultimate price for God and country. Today's civilian First Responders (police and firefighters) also take an oath to serve and protect our communities here at home.

The relationship between motorcycles and the law enforcement and military communities dates back to the earliest days of the twentieth century. Detroit, Michigan and Evanston, Illinois became the first cities to purchase a motorcycle for its police departments in 1908. Personally owned motorcycles were used as early as 1909

in Portland, Oregon, and Chief August Vollmer has been historically credited for the creation of the first official police motorcycle
patrol for the Berkeley Police Department in 1911.

Motorcycle enthusiasm has existed since the invention of the
first commercially available motorcycle and the moment any brave
individual with a heartbeat straddles one. In earnest, this enthusiasm predates the invention of the wheel. There is a genetic predis-
position for all humans to master their environment and their very
lives. From antiquity, man's desire to discover what's over the next
horizon has fueled the necessity to travel. The gasoline-fueled iron
horse replaced the grass-fed horse and helped usher in a new age
of travel, and with that, freedom. Necessity is the mother of invention, and today's motorcycle is the culmination of over a hundred
years of progress toward the ultimate of state-of-the-art engineer-
ing in personal ground transportation. Nothing offers the freedom of open-air travel like a motorcycle.

For the motorcycle enthusiast, it can be said that four wheels
may move our body, but two wheels move our souls.

Motorcycle clubs have been around as long as the motorcycle.
Any worthwhile human activity has within its precepts a desire to
be shared. Motorcycling is no different, and it can be said the mere
activity of riding in and of itself is so wrought with excitement,
pleasure, and mental tranquility that its enthusiasts naturally bond
with commonality across all differences in race, creed, and socio-
economic classes.

In 2001, four police officers from the Corpus Christi,
Texas Police Department shared such a bond and founded the
REGULADORE LEMC. Ron "Z-Man" Zirbes, Richard "Max"
Maxwell, Curtis Shelton, and Ed Longoria love riding and share
the brotherhood of military service, law enforcement, and their
enthusiasm for motorcycling. Inspired by their sheer will and
example of selfless sacrifice for their community, others sought
out affiliation and a nation-wide movement was born.

These four men founded not only a motorcycle club but also a brother and sisterhood that has continued to grow across the country with chapters that reach from coast to coast and from Canada to Mexico.

The Reguladores LEMC was founded, in their desire to share their love of motorcycling and to benefit the community of all citizens through charitable works. To this end, the Reguladores LEMC has raised and donated a fortune to charities across the United States.

I first rode my father's motorcycle and earned my license endorsement about two years after acquiring my driver's license in 1974. I was introduced to motor officer riding by Sgt. Phil Edmundson. By the time I had met Phil, I personally had been riding about twenty years. I approached him as he was leaving his shift on his motor and expressed my desire to ride with him some-time. Up to that point, I thought no I truly believed I knew how to ride. I was in for a rude awakening, as I quickly found out there was a whole new level to riding a motorcycle to its limits. I credit Phil for introducing police motor officer techniques and his assistance in getting me to motor training in 1995.

My personal involvement with Reguladores LEMC came about in 2009. I was riding with fellow military patriots Bob Weber and Kevin White, traveling together with our military colors proudly displayed. I was working with the East Carondelet Police Dept. with fellow officer Kevin White at the time. I had discussed rid-ing with a police motorcycle club, but I was dismayed at how little actual riding was done by local LEMCs.

Kevin, Bob, and I routinely did several Iron Butt rides annually, riding from Southern Illinois to Northern Wisconsin to Bike Week in Florida, to Rolling Thunder in DC, and to California and Texas.

All this was about to change when I was introduced to social media and a thing called Facebook in 2009. One day, I saw a pro-file picture of Tim Fulcher, a Madison County Sheriff's Dept.

member wearing a cut that caused me to stop and zoom in. This was the first time I saw Reguladores LEMC. I immediately contacted Tim, who in turn introduced me to USA member Brian "Chief" Benardin. From that day forward, I knew who I wanted to ride with, who I wanted to share this club with, and who would be included in my family.

The top rocker on our cuts says it all. We are friends with a shared history of service, we are friends who possess a love of riding motorcycles, we are friends who have become brothers and sisters through shared community service and charity, and we are friends who have become family.

WE ARE REGULADORES!

R. F. F. R.

Denzel D. Jines, II.

President, Southern Illinois Chapter, Reguladores.

CHAPTER 12

RANDOM THOUGHTS—REGULADORES LEMC

NATIONALS AFTERTHOUGHTS, AND WHY I

RIDE

Riding offers the participants the opportunity to experience freedom as symbolized by the wings on our cut. Freedom comes in many ways, and one of those freedoms is that during the time one rides, the ride becomes the entire focus of each and every participant. This time focusing on riding gives the rider's mind much needed rest, which heals one from all other mental stressors. Many can attest to how refreshed they feel after a truly physically and mentally demanding ride. They can finish a project or offer a solution that eluded them prior to the ride.

Many cannot participate due to health, age, or job-related issues that preclude the opportunity to do so. For them, the National party and other club activities become their focus, and they contribute immeasurably to the positive outcomes of all the backstage functioning and are essential to our club's success while forgoing the ride.

Throughout my riding life, I've been assaulted with comments by physicians calling my scoot a "donor cycle." I've heard, "You are crazy to risk XYZ." I've heard, "It's too hot, too cold, too this, too that. And the weather. Think of the bad weather." I took exception to one comment this weekend when someone wrote that an individual flying into the event was doing the "smart" thing to avoid the heat. I will reiterate there are legitimate reasons like medical, family, job, and time constraints that don't allow people to fully participate in this cherished activity of riding, but comfort is not one.

This is a motorcycle club. We ride motorcycles. I've belonged to plane clubs and car clubs and either flown or driven my particular toy to the respective event. Again, I reiterate, there are reasons people can't, and I'd wager they would prefer to ride if the circumstances could be changed. For those of us capable and WILLING, we plan for the riding conditions, we execute our plans, and we ride the ride no matter what obstacles fate places before us. It's SMART to ride. It takes smarts to preplan and prepare.

Enough rant.

CHAPTER 13

RANDOM THOUGHTS—ALS FUNDRAISER

"ARREST ALS" 2018

This is exactly what Regulardores LEMC is all about. "ARREST ALS."

Great events don't happen without a lot of blood, sweat, and tears, plus a few hurt feelings, some swearing, and occasional yelling, but if everyone puts their big-kid pants on, it works out. The time from inception to the event was one month. Great events require great planning.

Tonight, after a day of installing new custom wood shades and additional outdoor cafe lighting in solitude, I enjoy the company of friends that are family as they plan the final details of next week's Reguladores LEMC ALS fundraiser for the St. Louis ALS Foundation. Everyone was so serious and business-like, and I felt oddly out of sync. Several years ago, a book titled *Don't Sweat the Small Stuff . . . and It's All Small Stuff* was a best seller and I tried to take it to heart.

What if you knew your time was limited? What if today was your last? Questions like these reverberate inside my head daily as a reminder of that book's lessons. Every one of us will be dead soon enough. Everyone taking the time to read this will be dead in a hundred years.

As an ALS patient, I look at that diagnosis as a gift. It reminds me constantly that time is short. Don't waste it. Don't sweat the small stuff. Knowing this lesson and given my future (I'm a doctor so I fully understand the complexities of this situation) as an ALS patient, I felt out of sync with my friends as they were so serious while I was just content being with my friends and not overly worried about the details, club dynamics, personalities that are clashing, etc. Reguladores LEMC will put on a great fundraiser, and everything that can go wrong will, or it won't; however, it will be a great fundraiser nonetheless.

I would encourage even my healthiest friend to stop worrying about stuff, because you, just like me, are dying. I might get hit by a bus tomorrow, or you by a meteor. There are no guarantees. I think I'll just enjoy my company and not sweat anything tonight.

"ARREST ALS" was a fundraiser event that from inception to fruition was four short weeks. This event sponsored by the Southern Illinois Chapter of Reguladores LEMC and benefited the ALS Foundation of St. Louis. It raised over $6,000. This event saw the inauguration of the "Reguladores LEMC Annual Spirit Award."

The award is named after

Sgt. Albert Leal and Dr. Denzel Jines. Albert and I were both diagnosed with ALS, and the award was the club's honor to Al and myself. The award is given to a member who exhibits and personifies honor, integrity, character, and service.

Sgt. Leal was a police officer who served the Corpus Christi Texas for almost thirty years. Albert followed his own father's career path, Albert Sr., as a patrol officer, SWAT officer, and teacher, and was a distinguished leader amongst his peers. Albert was a two-time champion Golden Gloves boxer, who also won several Toughman Competitions, appearing on TV, as well as a body-builder and health advocate.

Albert was stricken with ALS in October 2016 and was taken from us in March 2018. Albert fought this disease to the end and never wavered in his faith or determination to beat this dreaded condition. He continued to ride right up to three weeks before his death.

The first recipient for this year's award was Bob Weber. Bob has been my cross-country Iron Butt (1000 miles in 24 hours) riding partner six times in the past three decades. Bob lives with the true Biker Spirit and can be counted upon to do the right thing when no one is watching. Bob has been the most tireless worker behind the scenes at every event he travels to, not just his own home events. Wherever and whenever there is a call for work, be it a friend moving, construction projects, or emergency aid, Bob is always the first to volunteer and the last to leave. This US Marine has lived the motto "First In" in every aspect of his life and has a reputation as a man of integrity and character. It was with this in mind that he was picked as the first recipient of what is now our club's most prestigious award.

My heartfelt thanks to all who worked for this event and for all who donated their hard-earned financial support. Mere words cannot express my gratitude for you all . . . Thank you.

The ALS charity event was for me a wonderful opportunity to see not only my Reguladores family but my Law Enforcement family, my Chiefs Dale Warke and Michael Dennis, and former partner Joe C. Paulfrey, as well as my brother Mark Jines. I have surrounded myself with men of integrity and character and consider myself most fortunate in keeping company with such men.

I was touched right in the feels, having a memorial award named after Albert and me and then see it given to a close friend. I think I am going to try to make more memories before I make my final farewells. Neither Albert nor myself are or were defined by ALS and as always seized the day.

The following is about one of the posters produced for an ad for the event.

Arrest ALS Raffle Post

To all my FB friends, I am selling raffle tickets for a wheelbarrow full of top-shelf liquor. If you love a quaffable libation and like good odds please, buy a few tickets. Even better, just please donate to this event. All proceeds go to the St. Louis ALS Foundation. As a healthcare provider, I have personally witnessed the work this organization does. As a patient, I have benefitted from their care. Every penny of this current event will go to provide direct care in the St. Louis area. I am also asking anyone who is within an hour or two drive and who would like to come to talk with me that day and give to something that will truly be appreciated by someone in true need please come by that day.

CHAPTER 14

RANDOM THOUGHTS—FLYING WWII WARBIRDS (MY LAST FLIGHT AS PILOT IN CHARGE)

I've loved aviation since being introduced to flight as a young boy. My first models besides Julie Newmar and Raquel Welch were . . . no, no, nope, not those models. My first models were WWII planes like B-17, P-51, Zero and M-109s, and today, I have autographs of original Flying Tiger aviators Chuck Yeager and Dick Cole, who were pioneers of aviation and heroes from the Greatest Generation. Their collective stories were an inspiration for me to earn a pilot's license and fly a few WWII warbirds.

My wife purchased a great birthday present for me, and yesterday, I took full advantage of the great weather and flew the WWII advanced training fighter plane, the A6 Texan N97VR, and put her through the paces doing some air combat maneuvers in the skies over central Illinois. I haven't flown this plane in fifteen years, and as a former pilot, I felt rusty. Kevin Kegan, who was my flight instructor, nursed me through the first few rolls as the training started to come back, and now it's Monday, and I have a little surgery to do on my friend and tattoo artist (got to pay for the next Vitamin Ink injection, you know).

Darla, thank you for thinking of this experience, because I had all but given up flying, thinking those days are over. I could no longer use my right foot to input enough right rudder to overcome P factor during high angle (oh, sorry about the tech talk). I love you and appreciate you so much. This was something that always made me feel young, alive, and almost as good as a kiss.

CHAPTER 15

RANDOM THOUGHTS—HEALTH IS OUR MOST PRECIOUS ASSET, AND HOW TO GET RICH SLOWLY

There are, in these United States, currently nine million millionaires. The vast majority of these people share several common characteristics. They stayed married to the same spouse for over fifty years. They live below their means in the same house they purchased as newlyweds. They never earned more than $17,000 in a given year. What?! That's right, $17,000 a year. So, you may ask, how did they do it? They saved small amounts of every paycheck for their entire lives. They started small and grew it big.

You could be the wealthiest person on the planet in terms of financial wealth, but without your health, you possess a rather poor quality of life.

Sylvester Stallone, Arnold Schwarzenegger, Chuck Norris are all well past their prime and in their seventies, yet are still in the game. They are currently the exception to the rule, but I truly believe they are what could and should be the norm. Just because 90 percent of the population has gum disease, heart disease, obesity, etc. doesn't make that normal. It is usual but not normal. These guys are what should pass for normal.

So, what do these examples have to do with living with ALS? Everything! There are no treatments for ALS that are curative. Common sense dictates that the healthier the host, the longer it will take any disease entity to produce a loss of function. Lifestyle is thus more important to anyone handed a catastrophic diagnosis like ALS.

Neither of these examples were born models of fitness nor anatomically ready to pose for a statue by Da Vinci, let alone ready for a close up for Mr. DeMille (Sunset Blvd reference). They worked at it over time. They invested in their health.

Modern medicine treats disease. You must be the one who becomes your own best advocate for your health. Modern prescription medicines, for the most part, treats symptoms but do not cure the underlying cause. Most meds are like spraying a flowery potpourri in a toilet. Poopy flowers wafting gently into one's nostrils isn't as appealing a proposition as flowers by themselves. I digress . . .

It is far better to remove the illness than just covering up the symptoms.

Your health begins and ends with you and not your doctor. Diet and exercise are the keys to health. A healthy lifestyle is far more important than who your doctor is or what meds you are ordered to take. My goal is to take no medications or at least the fewest meds necessary to survive. I want my patients and myself to exit this life much like a light switch operates instead of dying a piece at a time with amputations, sick from the side effects of all the meds we take, ED, blind on dialysis . . .

A healthy lifestyle is our best start toward a better, longer life. Just like getting rich, we do it slow daily and consistently. It won't cure ALS, but it will make it harder for ALS to get the job done.

CHAPTER 16

RANDOM THOUGHTS—DENTAL HEALTH RELATES TO OVERALL GENERAL HEALTH

In this chapter, let's look at dental health. Your dental health can be an asset or a nidus of systemic illness. That's right. Your teeth can make your whole body sick. If you have ALS, your oral hygiene must be kept up in order to decrease your chances of increasing overall inflammation that accelerates the loss of antioxidants and therefore increasing the speed with which ALS may progress.

Dentistry in a Nutshell: How We Practice Oral Medicine at Southampton Dental.
During any given day in practice, we treated dental issues ranging from a traumatized tongue which was referred by one of my physician colleagues, to removal of teeth on a patient referred from another dental provider, to treating and restoring dental caries (cavities) and periodontal (gum) disease.

We fielded questions on issues ranging from patients' concerns about how they got dental disease to how their medical conditions are related. I discussed the risks of a particular procedure with a physician regarding the use of bone-strengthening drugs and also whether or not this patient may need to discontinue anticoagulant therapy. His opinion was that it is my call since I was the one doing the surgery.

One common theme in practice, whether it be dentistry or medicine, is the amount of time we spend treating chronic preventable illness. A good ballpark number is that the USA spends roughly 70 percent of its healthcare dollars on chronic, oft preventable illnesses. In dentistry, we often spend a great deal of clinic time redoing previously placed dental restorations (not ones I've placed!); in other words, redoing or replacing old dental work

The insurance industry loves collecting premiums but is reluctant to pay for needless dental or medical procedures. Given this reluctance, wouldn't you find it odd that these same insurance companies willingly pay (albeit begrudgingly) for a dentist to replace a filling only two years old or a crown that's only five years old? They do. Insurance companies use actuarial tables and complicated algorithms to determine risks, etc., and they have deemed it is legitimate to pay for these procedures. This reality suggests there are a significant number of restoration failures or recurring dental decay to warrant this expenditure.

The dental materials I use in my practice to restore teeth will outlast the cockroaches. Gold, silver, ceramics, and composites (plastic) materials last thousands of years. So why do I have to replace fillings etc., especially when the current literature is replete with examples of restorations utilizing these materials lasting twenty to eighty years?

The answer we have found is a combination of ignorance coupled with a lack of personal motivation. But how can a patient be motivated if they are woefully uninformed about their own condition?

Dental disease is caused by bacteria or bacterial plaque. That white film you can scrape off for a tooth is plaque and it's alive. Think of it as a bug. These microbes have great big names like *Streptococcus mutans* and *Porphyromonas gingivalis*, but as the term microbe implies, they are very small. There are approximately 750 morphologically and biochemically different species of "bug" that grow in the human mouth. Some of these critters eat the sugar and foods that you eat and in turn eat you.

"But Doctor, I thought weak teeth run in my family. Weak gums too. Everyone in my family has dentures." These are real quotes from patients.

Myths die hard and doctors must break down barriers built of misinformation in order to educate patients that don't know what they don't know!

About four years ago, the Annals of Internal Medicine published work on the physical expression of genetically linked illnesses. The analysis of years of the literature demonstrated close to 90 percent of all these genetic disorders required an environmental trigger. So, to answer my patients' inquiries as to how they developed dental disease, I tell them the only part of the majority of dental diseases that runs in almost any family is your grandparents didn't tell your parents, who in turn didn't tell you, how to prevent the easiest preventable yet most commonly occurring illness in all of mankind: brush and floss (or better yet, water floss).

Did you know that bleeding gums and chronic dental infections are an independent risk factor for heart disease and stroke? It is not a coincidence that the plaque on your teeth and the artery-clogging plaque that can stop your heart have the same name. How about that? The most commonly suffered disease and the most common cause of death are truly linked.

Okay, so how does one go about preventing cavities and other dental maladies? Brushing and flossing are the basics. Rinsing with anti-microbial rinses like Listerine to kill bacteria helps as well. I might even prescribe prescription toothpaste.

A few of my patients can actually use a manual toothbrush to adequately remove enough plaque to prevent cavities. Most patients that use a manual brush manage to utilize them for an average of approximately thirty seconds at a time. This is about a quarter of the amount of time we recommend brushing one time. We recommend you brush two to three times a day, and even more in some cases. The average patient brushes too hard with their hard-bristled brush and, combined with a minty toothpaste, they assume they are tingly and minty fresh. In reality though, they are not thoroughly clean.

We recommend a modern electric toothbrush like Sonicare or Oral B. These brushes not only scrub teeth up to a thousand times per second, they have built-in computer chips that keep them running for a full two minutes, which is the bare minimum amount of time necessary to adequately remove all the plaque and create a healthy oral environment.

What about the space between the teeth? You know, the other two sides of your teeth that only get cleaned when food gets stuck there. Floss. Floss. Floss. Even better, water flossing after flossing. Why? It's just like a row of houses, and all the front and back yards get mowed. No one ever mows between the houses. Obviously, that's where the weeds first grow, the junk accumulates, and finally, termites and rats start living there. You have to clean up the area between the houses. Same goes for teeth.

So, how do you clean between teeth, and what's the best way?

Think about changing a baby's diaper and accidentally getting your fingers . . . um . . . yucky. Simply wiping them off with a tissue or paper towel removes the graphic evidence that you had poo on your fingers. However, they would not make you sanitary or ready to handle food. Wiping floss between the teeth helps like the tissue at getting off the larger amount of contamination like food debris. However, all the chemicals, toxins, and nasty stuff produced by the bacteria are still there. For your hands, we recommend soap and water, and for your teeth, unless you cuss a lot, try Listerine and pressure washing with a water flosser to remove bacteria and diluting all the chemicals and bacterial waste out. The solution to pollution, in this case, is dilution. The washing spray removes and dilutes the end byproducts of the bacteria's metabolism: enzymes that destroy tissue, acids, and bacterial endotoxins, etc.

The way dentistry works in my practice is that no matter where we start with a particular patient, we can get them to a highly functional esthetic dentition. Our goal is to get a patient, through a means of combined education (the term doctor means teacher) and treatment to as healthy dentition as possible, and most importantly, to *remain so.*

A healthy lifestyle is our best start toward a better, longer life.

CHAPTER 17

RANDOM THOUGHTS—WHERE DENTISTRY

INTERSECTS WITH MEDICINE

All ALS patients should seek preventive and corrective care to minimize the systemic manifestation of oral diseases.

Acid Erosion and the Intersection between Dentistry and Medicine

Here is a case (not the bulimia we were taught about in dental but the more commonly seen) that hopefully everyone recognizes and can relate to. This short Pearl Note is about not how we treat this dentally. There are several right ways to approach this. This is about something far more common that most clinicians know and things to think about when we see it.

During routine dental exams, I conduct a review of systems after going over their health questionnaire, past medical history, their chief complaint, current medications, social history, their history of present illness, etc., I ask, "Do you have any pain, burning, belching, heartburn, ringing in the ears, blurry or double vision, any lumps or bumps or pimples that don't seem to go away?" Okay, what does this have to do with acid erosion?

Any patient that presents with acid erosion and has a history of burning, belching, and heartburn requires a work up for an infection, a tumor, or GERD, which is acid reflux or regurgitation. Rule out the zebras first in an upper GI series and special radiographs of the stomach to rule out a stomach tumor that accounts for much less than 1 percent chance in the cases we see. Blood testing for a bacteria called *Helicobacter pylori* is usually done today as it has been shown to cause the vast majority of stomach ulcers and reflux symptoms. *Helicobacter pylori* can be treated with antibiotics, and there are several protocols for treating your patients, even if the blood test is negative, because there are at least two dozen other species of bacteria and viruses that cause ulcers and reflux that are not detected on simple blood screenings. Big work ups with the patient's primary care physician usually lead to a referral to a gastroenterologist who will perform endoscopy of the stomach, where a biopsy is done with reported nebulous results. In other words, there are many false negatives with this testing. Often because of the limitations in laboratory medicine, we end up with a diagnosis or GERD. Treatment for GERD is lifelong and only covers up the symptoms. This is the unfortunate part of medicine where a patient gets a diagnosis whose meaning is that you have pain and dysfunction, and we will give it a name like GERD or fibromyalgia or osteoarthritis, because we don't know why.

I was fortunate as a resident to meet an attending physician and research fellow who would later earn the Nobel Prize in medicine for his discovery of the etiology of stomach ulcers . . . you know the burning, belching, heartburn. Barry Marshal, MD discovered this in 1983 by a rather unorthodox method of inoculating himself with *Helicobacter*. He then suffered the slings and arrows of conventional medicine that never let progress get in the way of tradition. He was told that that's not how we treat ulcers here . . . ulcers are caused by emotional stress, spicy foods, your own immune system waking up Monday morning and deciding to attack your own stomach. It was later reported that just like HPV was associated with cervical cancer, *H. pylori* was associated with stomach cancer.

There are several strains (hundred) of *Helicobacter—pylori, rappini, helmanni*—so along with other bacteria and viruses like CMV that have been shown to cause ulcers, which in turn cause acid reflux, which in turn erodes teeth (had to bring this back to dentistry). However, there are limitations to testing for the cause of the symptoms we see as burning, belching, and heartburn. Large medical centers have access to PCR testing, which is expensive, that help definitively diagnose which of these are the cause, but for the most part, our patients are seldom worked up for this, and so the most widely prescribed medicines today are for the symptoms instead of the cure, which is a short course of antibiotics! I even prescribed the antibiotics in the face of negative labs! The reasoning is in the literature, large numbers of false-negative testing being one.

We are lucky in dental medicine that we can see the cause and treat it empirically with a myriad of products in a plethora of different procedures to fix our patient's dental needs, sometimes permanently. There are many in medicine who treat the symptoms of the patient's chief complaint to the standard of care yet miss the cause. This later translates to further morbidity in our patients and potential mortality, as cancers can develop from untreated causes.

I always consult with the patients' primary care physician, informing them of my clinical findings and that I would like them worked up for infection with *H. pylori*. If they are lucky enough to have a good physician who finds this particular germ, it can be easily eradicated with one or two separate courses of antibiotics. There are some resistant strains of *H. pylori*, so if the symptoms return or a second titer shows an active infection, then we can follow a second antibiotic protocol for treatment.

By looking at not just the teeth but at the patient as a whole, you may save them from a lifetime of meds that cause other iatrogenically-induced illnesses, cancer, and, more importantly for dentists, further acid erosion that requires retreatment.

ALS patients cannot afford to suffer from dental disease. The effects of dental disease can increase oxidative stress on a system already stressed.

CHAPTER 18

RANDOM THOUGHTS—DIABETES AND

DENTISTRY

I posted this on the clinical website *Dental Clinical Pearls* as food for thought about our health.

Dentistry and Diabetes: Not Our Patients but Us
ALS patients develop comorbidities. It's tough enough to have ALS, so eliminating any additional illnesses (comorbidities) can help ALS patients.

Anyone can benefit from this advice, especially if you are an ALS patient. There are pearls in this essay I originally wrote for dentists that an ALS patient can use to decrease their overall levels of systemic inflammation.

Dentistry is a stressful, physically demanding profession; however, the physically demanding part is in its health-destroying sedentary nature and not in its vigorous demand like being a CrossFit instructor. Yes, many of us run up and down the hall from one operatory to another, but never should a dentist accept the delusion that this constitutes real exercise. We should never live on the laurels of our high school and college athletic careers, as evidenced by Al Bundy.

Diabetes is a leading cause of blindness, amputations, heart disease (insulin resistance can predict heart disease), kidney failure, impotence. Millions of Americans have been diagnosed, and millions more suffer without the benefit of diagnosis. We are (the vast majority) genetically programmed to become diabetics, as diabetics are better capable of withstanding long periods of famine. Dentists are not immune to this disease and need to understand we can cure early-onset diabetes if we recognize it in ourselves, and we can then be better stewards to our patients.

Medical literature is replete with examples of how even short periods (two weeks) of physical inactivity can cause muscle atrophy, increased weakness, increased insulin resistance, and increased body fat, driving up post-prandial glucose levels. (Diabetologia, Jun 2018;61(6):1282-1294, J Gerontol A Biol Sci Med Sci, Jul 9, 2018;73(8):1070–1077).

The mechanism for how blood sugar levels rise and in turn increase body fat, which in turn increases insulin resistance, which then leads to increased post-prandial glucose spikes that cause neurological damage when the extra sugar sticks to nerves and converts to a neurotoxin sorbitol increasing oxidative stress on nerves because the fat-laden insulin receptors are incapable of responding, thereby increasing potentials for huge insulin dumps that increase the population hunger drive that then makes the individual eat even more food that drives the sugar levels beyond the muscle's and liver's storage capacity until even more triglycerides are formed to store the excess sugars as fat that sticks to insulin receptors . . . the bottom line here is increased muscle mass increases one's ability to store sugar for energy better than fat and makes one less insulin resistant.

I purposely wrote that very long run-on sentence to get us thinking about the complexity that sugar metabolism encompasses and its absolute responsibility in the etiology of metabolic syndrome X and adult-onset diabetes.

With all this, we haven't even touched on the inflammatory aspect of this condition and the effects of Short Chain Fatty Acids (SCFA) and how the trillions of bacteria (we cause huge effects daily with prescribing antibiotics) in our bodies control digestion, immunity, etc. . . . I am getting ahead of myself, here.

I have said this before and recommend to my patients that they all should exercise and eat a more plant-based diet.

Studies published in Annals of Internal Medicine several years ago and just this year (Scand J Med Sci Sports, Mar 2018;28(3):1048–1055) indicate lifestyle can trump (not the politician) genes. There are actually new studies in epigenetics showing how lifestyle changes can affect (modify) DNA and either turn on or turn off genes. Seventy percent of healthcare dollars are spent on lifestyle preventable illnesses. One-half of the medicines prescribed in this country are written to control the side effects of medicines taken by patients for the treatment of illnesses that could be controlled through a healthy diet and adequate exercise.

So, here are a few recommendations that will help us all get on track so we can reduce morbidity in ourselves and thereby practice our passion for dentistry on a high level.

Research for more than seventy years has shown the benefits of eating a plant-based diet, and the results are finally being explained in a manner that makes recommendations easier with a firm footing in real science. Individuals on a heavily weighted plant-based diet have more short-chain fatty acids available, which reduce inflammation, help to lower high levels of blood sugar and cholesterol, and even help with increasing intestinal mucous, which is beneficial in controlling gut flora balance. Patients with higher levels of SCFAs have better-modulated immunity and reduced inflammation, which in turn decreases the risk of heart disease, diabetes, colon cancer, and even obesity. Eat a wide variety of plants, especially green, dark-colored veggies and fruits, whole grains, high fiber foods, beans, seeds, and nuts, and stay away from fruit juices and added sugars, artificial sweeteners, and excess red meats (shown to increase diabetes). Start strength training to increase muscle mass. Cardio like running and cycling are great for the heart but lack the benefit of increasing muscle mass as fast or as efficiently as resistance training.

Nutrients, 2011 Oct; 3(10): 858–876. Science, Mar 9, 2018:359(6380):1151–1156, Diabetes Care, July 2008, Epidem Reviews, Jan 1, 1993;15(2):499–545, Mutat Res, Jul–Aug 2009;682(1):39–53, Cancer Discov, Dec, 2014;4(12):1387–1397, Diabetes, 2009 Jul; 58(7):1509–1517, J Lipid Res, Sep 2013;54(9):2325–40.American Journal of Epidemiology, Dec 1, 1987;126(6):1093–1102, Nutrition Journal, July 10, 2018;17:67.

CHAPTER 19

RANDOM THOUGHTS—CAREER PATH FOR

GENERAL DENTISTS

After my diagnosis with ALS, I was still active in dental practice and education, and after retirement, I've remained involved in education and training.

One way I pay back my profession is to educate younger doctors. This can be by answering clinical questions or more universal questions about our field, its place in medicine, and even business.

Any business questions I refer to my office manager of thirty years, Katherine Weyhaupt. She has a business degree and has been instrumental in creating relationships with hospitals, federal, and state and local health agencies that put Southampton Dental at the forefront of Dental and Oral Medicine. We are all very proud of her daughter, Michelle Weyhaupt. Valedictorian, perfect SAT, Cum Laude at Alabama, highest possible MCAT score, medical school at Vanderbilt. She certainly took after her mother.

In this world of specialization, it behooves young general dentists to seek as much additional training as possible in order to meet the demands of a more sophisticated patient population. There are several worthwhile post-doctoral training avenues open, and each has a specific value when creating your own private practice.

AEGDs are great for those interested in seeking further expertise in specific disciplines. If you are fortunate enough to join the military, most of the practicing career dental officers are board-certified in either an ADA approved specialty or a recognized Federal Dental Specialty (Operative, Oral Med, Comp Dentists . . . You were most likely trained by one or more of these).

Federal Dental Specialty in Comprehensive Dentistry is a three-year residency at Bethesda Maryland. General dentists complete rotations under the supervision of specialists in each discipline, including much of the didactic reading of the other specialists. This training is designed to put a dentist into an area where he may not have specialists to back him up and he must therefore be able to handle cases that are complex usually requiring one or more specialists. Graduates of this program are eligible for the Certifying Board in General Dentistry and the Federal Services Board that recognizes these graduates for increased federal specialty pay and benefits.

GPRs will acquaint dentists with where their field intersects with medicine and get them ready to work in a hospital setting. Students in GPRs are encouraged to join the Special Needs Dentistry organization and take Fellowship exams (Hospital Dentistry) and even Board Certification in Special Needs Dentistry (DABSND).

The Academy of General Dentistry offers certification of most of the continuing education you receive upon graduation and is the voice of general dentists. It offers a Fellowship Award (FAGD) after you complete more than three hundred hours of CEs, with the majority being participatory classes and taking their Fellowship Exam, which is a day-long written exam covering everything you should know about general dentistry. After completing eight hundred hours, you can earn the Mastership Award in General Dentistry (MAGD). These honors are designed to distinguish those who are current and seeking continuing education on a steady basis.

Every one of these avenues and others allow practitioners a means to differentiate themselves from their peers while earning respected credentials recognized not only by their peers but their patients.

D. D. Jines, DMD, MD, FAAHD, FAGD, MAGD, DABSND ret.

I never put all this alphabet soup out, but this seems like a good time.

CHAPTER 20

RANDOM THOUGHTS—NEW GRADUATES

I started writing short pieces for *Dental Clinical Pearls*, a continuing education website prior to retirement but well after my diagnosis with ALS. This particular essay offers insight that a layperson can use to ask their dentist questions about training, and that is why I have included many of these.

A new doctor graduates having completed the basic requirements for their doctoral degree. For many in various fields of healthcare, this is the beginning of their education as they then specialize in narrower fields of focus.

Upon graduation, where a new doctor has just weeks prior required supervision, general practitioners are thrust into an uncomfortable role of being the expert in the room.

General family practitioners are thrust into a gatekeeper primary care role that requires the understanding not only of their own limitations but also advanced techniques in several of the specialties areas.

In medicine, a plastic surgeon can further specialize in hand surgery or breast reconstruction, while a general surgeon may advertise as a cosmetic surgeon doing breast augmentation and a gynecologist may perform cosmetic vaginal surgeries. General dentists perform a plethora of procedures that encompass every aspect of dentistry and every specialty. They should be held to the same clinical standards of care when providing procedures that specialty dentists perform. A well-trained general dentist should be able to provide endodontic treatment of a tooth indistinguishable from the same treatment performed by an endodontist, otherwise why do the treatment at all. Exodontia is NOT oral surgery. Every dentist should be able to remove the teeth. The list of procedures goes on and on, and what I want to address to the young, NEW doctors is training after dental school.

Everyone desires admiration and respect. It's a basic human trait. General practitioners can gain a sense of purpose and pride when performing vital services patients truly need. Confidence can be gained through clinical excellence that is achieved through professionally recognized training programs, residency, mentorship, and the desire to improve the level of care you provide thereby improving the quality of your practice and your own life.

Side Note: If you do great dentistry, you will have decreased stress and a better life, and you'll be able to sleep with a clean conscience.

High quality continuing education will illustrate what truly excellent clinical work can and should look like. Dentists make the clinical determination of what is clinically acceptable by what they have personally seen. If a dentist has not had the benefit of seeing true operative dental masters creating lifelike anatomically correct teeth, they will settle for and accept block chiclet-like restorations worthy of the scorn heaped upon them by their clinical betters.

Anyone who has read my posts understands I never speak unkindly about another dentist to a patient. I never throw another dentist under the bus. I do discuss poor quality, clinically unacceptable work with colleagues. I will testify in court about what standards of care were missed, etc.; however, for the most part, I don't or won't speak poorly of another. I wasn't there.

General dentists should join the Academy of General Dentistry, for starters. It is the organization that actually fights for you. Next, seek Fellowship then Mastership then Board Certification in General Dentistry. Go to Pankey, join study groups, check out CRA and Gordon Christensen, read JADA, triple O, JPD at a minimum monthly. These are steps general dentists can take to be recognized as a leader in our chosen field and increase our clinical abilities to outstanding levels of quality only rivaled by specialists, and in many cases even better.

D. D. Jines, DMD, MD

Fellow Academy of General Dentistry and American Association of Hospital Dentists, Mastership Academy of General Dentistry, Diplomate American Board of Special Needs Dentistry (retired)

CHAPTER 21

RANDOM THOUGHTS—PATIENT DIALOGUE

After reading this Random Thought, an ALS patient and caregiver should be able to open a dialogue with their dental healthcare provider to improve and maintain their dental health.

Patient dialogues to communicate an office philosophy based on excellence, preventive care, and long-term success should be taught to students, as words have the power to heal or kill. That is true, whether we are talking able patients, children, or even within ourselves.

Learning how to talk to a patient can build relationships with even the most difficult people. It can prevent a malpractice suit better than the actual beauty and quality of your restorative work.

New dentists, please don't expect patients to trust or even respect you right off the bat. You just graduated, and that means you've accomplished the basic minimum requirements necessary to be called Doctor. Today's world distrusts our profession more than it did thirty years ago. For all our new patients know, you got into this because you can make money. You may sell any treatment just to make a buck. There is an ongoing court case where an oncologist has been accused of falsely diagnosing cancer so he could prescribe meds that he received kickbacks on.

Learning to talk and build relationships will get your expensive procedures treatment planned and accepted without the "sales" dialogue some would have you buy. Yes, you are, in many instances, competing with new color TV and kitchen rehab ala' Chip and Joanna on Fixer Upper. You don't have to compete when the patients know you have their best interests in mind.

I just talk on these instructional videos extemporaneously. We must remember even physicians, nurses, lawyers, etc. know nada, zilch, almost nothing about teeth and dentistry. Keep it simple! I've had patients blame their last dentist—that's you and me—for discomfort in a tooth after it was FIXED. I explain how inflammation works the same way in a finger or a tooth without breaking down mast cells, bradykinins, prostaglandins, etc. I explain teeth are joints and can become sprained or strained, and just like a knee or hip, may require being replaced. Teeth, just like any tissue that's been operated on, may let us know that it's going to rain tomorrow (baralgia). I tell patients about our practice philosophy and why hygiene is so important. This is rudimentary yet needs to be said.

Thoughts on Explaining Plaque
It's alive. I tell patients it's "sugar bugs." Literally, it is something that eats what we eat, and then eats us. It's no coincidence that dental plaque shares the same name as the stuff that blocks our arteries. I even remind MDs of all the literature that references the tie ins to oral plaque and the plaque that blocks our arteries.

Flossing and Dentistry 101
The following is my personal take on the controversy about flossing and things to think about in the wonderful world of teeth . . . basically, this is what I told every patient who is welcomed into my clinic and the same is reiterated by my staff.

Now, since this is for general consumption, I will leave most of the scientific jargon out. These points hold true whether given to my neurosurgeon friends, nurses, any other healthcare provider, or the general public.

The way dentistry can work today is that no matter what a patient's condition is when they start to care, in my practice, we can go from fully bombed out mouth (gum disease, infections, missing teeth, cavities, abscesses, etc.) to ideally restored functioning dentition (gum care including surgery, extraction, fillings, crowns, bridges, implants).

The nice part about doing dentistry today is that the materials I use for restoring teeth (the same materials I've used for over thirty years) can last a lifetime. Gold, silver, ceramics, composites (think plastics) can last thousands of years, probably long enough that the only thing still surviving will be cockroaches.

The way modern dentistry works today is we examine a patient and determine if any treatment is necessary. Dental treatment, like many medical treatments, has a rhyme and reason for a certain order in which it is accomplished. The goal is to stop new damage, ensure the supporting structures are healthy and remain so, maybe remove hopeless teeth if needed, then fix those teeth in need of repair, and finally replace any missing teeth. When all of the planned treatment is completed, the only thing left should be seeing the patient every six months to ensure the patient is remaining healthy.

Imagine hiring a handyman to help you construct a new deck on your house, a really nice deck with composite decking and even a fireplace and water feature. However, while you are working on the deck, you notice the inside of the kitchen is on fire. If you continue deck construction and keep adding a new, fancy railing, it just wouldn't make any sense. Your priorities change, and you have to put out that fire, or everything you do will be for nothing. Right? That is why the first thing we do in my office is to teach every patient the importance of proper oral hygiene and how to maintain it. Only then can I hope to restore teeth and they stay restored for a lot longer than the average.

My goal when I restore a tooth is for that particular restoration to last the rest of the patient's life. In general, the insurance industry will pay me to restore the same tooth every two years . . . Think about that. The insurance industry loves to collect premiums and can find an infinite number of ways to delay a payment or even not pay for services contracted by the insured individual, but somehow, they are forced to pay to retreat a tooth over and over. This should give you pause to think that if they will pay for a tooth to be treated every couple of years, just how often do restored teeth actually fail in the real world? Why do these teeth require retreatment? What is causing all this dental disease?

According to current dental scientific literature, the cause of the dental disease is bacterial plaque (think tooth bugs). It is the white stuff that you can scrape off a tooth that crawls, if you are looking at it under a microscope. They have long names like *streptococcus mutans*. However, they are very tiny little living organisms that produce very nasty chemicals after they eat the sugar you eat, and then in turn they eat you or your teeth, which happen to be the hardest structure in your body.

I know that for those dentists that practice what we preach, we brush, floss, utilize rinses that are anti-microbial (kill bacteria, etc.), and therefore go throughout our lifetimes never requiring the type of care we ourselves render to patients. Dentists are seldom dental patients. Most dentists get their teeth fixed in dental school and learn how to prevent dental disease, which is the most common disease suffered by humankind.

What? Yes, dental disease, the most common malady suffered by all humans, is also one of the most preventable of all illnesses. It is important to note that the most common disease suffered by man is also related to the most common cause of death. It is kind of funny how that works. Dental disease is also associated with a plethora of other systemic illnesses, from infertility to low birth weight babies, asthma, strokes, and so forth. Now, let me get back on point.

If I am not a genetically enhanced super being (there is specu-
lation that I am the product of scientific experiments, but that's
for a later discussion), how is it I don't have any dental diseases?
I simply brushed and flossed with the technology at hand in my
twenties and thirties, and gradually increased the efficiency and
frequency of my oral hygiene as I aged and as dental hygiene tech-
nologies improved. Manual brushes were adequate and worked as
long as I was motivated and understood their proper use. Floss
helped disrupt the plaque between the teeth and Listerine helped
kill the remaining bacteria, so for thirty years, every time I sat in a
chair to get my teeth examined and cleaned, my hygienists would
look and say there's nothing they need do so I was free to go. My
goal was to get all my patients to that same level. The only difference between them and me was that I knew how to do it and why
to do it and was motivated to do it.

Today, we have enhanced electronic toothbrushes capable of
brushing a thousand strokes a second and timers that keep the brush
running the minimum amount of time I believe necessary to clean
all teeth, which is two minutes at least two times every day. We have
water flossers that research is showing removes more plaque than
string floss and additionally irrigates out not only the bacteria but
also the chemical soup the bacteria leave behind. It is this chemical
soup of acids, enzymes, and toxins that cause dental disease, either
directly or through a reaction with your body's immune system.

You should know that as a former instructor of plastic surgery, I
would scrub before surgery to essentially decrease the potential of
contaminating the operating field with bacteria that could possibly infect the patient and thereby cause unnecessary post-surgical
infection, scarring, or other complications, including even death.
We have safety protocols in my clinic and in every hospital, even
restaurants, etc. advising us to wash our hands and use all those
disinfectants to wipe down that remote control for the TV in the
hotel, yet now some guy is stating that flossing isn't necessary.

What about some common sense when it comes to reporting? Without getting into all the details of the recent article concerning flossing, suffice it to say there is a whole lot left out of this article and context is important. One needs to only apply a little common sense to understand that the demonstrated cause of the dental disease is bacteria. It accumulates on the teeth and should be removed every day. It has been demonstrated that when plaque (bugs) are removed correctly, the measurements of the severity of dental disease are decreased. The individual's systemic health is improved when plaque is removed and, again, this can be measured in a variety of ways. Inflammatory markers like CRP (C-Reactive Protein) are decreased.

When I treat my oncology patients receiving chemo or radiation therapy or organ transplant patients or joint replacement patients or cardiac patients or immune-suppressed patients, our collective goal is to decrease the incidence of systemic odontogenic infection (dental infections that have spread to distant body structures). We use every tool we have and in the past, string flossing was shown in our patient populations to be a necessary adjunct to tooth brushing as it was the only thing that effectively removed the germs from between the teeth.

While I still use string floss on occasion, I do recommend water flossing as a more effective alternative, in combination with electronic brushes like Sonicare and Oral B electric brushes. Over the past twenty years, patients utilizing these tools have remained free of caries and have avoided the need to return for restorative dental care or even more invasive surgical care.

That's my two cents for everyone on this topic, including ALS patients.

What an ALS patient can take from this particular essay is to have a dialogue with your doctors. Ask them what they would do. Ask them why. Ask them how.

CHAPTER 22

RANDOM THOUGHTS—MAINTAINING YOUR

CLINICAL EDGE

One of the best parts about the *Dental Clinical Pearls* site is seeing outstanding clinical performances that regularly augment the knowledge base of our youngest and newest members. For me, being able to seemingly remain relevant as ALS tries to steal my dexterity has been a great way to stave off depression.

There is not a single one best way to restore a patient. Unlike religion, there are several ways to restore a single tooth.

I never speak ill about others, even when it is really crappy work. I wasn't in that other dentist's office during that procedure. I don't have ALL the info, so downgrading others doesn't lift my clinical abilities. Training, continuing education, and especially participatory advanced training will lift your clinical abilities.

Every one of you has a clinical cut off as to what you deem as clinically acceptable. Dentistry runs the spectrum from quackery to textbook ideal. I have found that the more training I have received by high-end programs, the higher my clinical cut off is. Seeing great work here on this *Dental Clinical Pearls* page helps all of us make our clinical cut off to what we accept much higher than those who only get the bare minimum of continuing education.

I encourage residency training or associating with mentors who have "been there, done that" so as to avoid clinical disasters and to render advanced clinical care.

There is nothing more noble than general practice done on a textbook level. It has always puzzled me why there are so many specialties in medicine and dentistry. I understand from a didactic standpoint, but a clinical one . . . We have a specialty whose total amount of tissue would not fill a thimble (endodontics). They are experts on micro wound healing, yet the clinical practice even with microscopes shouldn't intimidate anyone from performing excellent root canal therapy. Exodontia is not a specialty, and every dentist should be able to remove any tooth

Note that I am not dissing ANY specialty!

Join the AGD, seek residency training, join study clubs, read, go to Panky, Gordon Christiansen. Make your clinical cut off higher by seeing better work.

I am not a specialist. I am a GP who did an AEGD, then two-year GPR, then earned Fellowship and Mastership in AGD and Fellowship in the American Association of Hospital Dentists, earning Diplomate Status in the American Board of Special Needs Dentistry, as well as earning a Medical degree and becoming faculty at a teaching hospital. There are programs to become board certified in General Dentistry, and the Federal Services recognize a specialty in Comprehensive General Dentistry after training like I mentioned above.

Instead of advertising and having a professional radio announcer say things like you are the best as you fight over crumbs, you could be building a strong growing practice without a need to advertise by expanding your clinical knowledge base and providing needed treatments instead padding a bill with production production production ultimately losing patients because they feel undervalued or overcharged.

So, yesterday, in our private practice, we had a referral for me to remove a large bilateral tori, endodontic treatment, and extractions of impacted wisdom teeth, in addition to doing hygiene and tooth restorations, etc.

Lesson to take away for dental students from this is short missive is to read on this site Dental Clinical Pearls as much and as often as possible and to expand your clinical knowledge.

CHAPTER 23

RANDOM THOUGHTS—ORAL CANCER

I was diagnosed with ALS before I was diagnosed with prostate cancer. My thoughts on oral cancer are relevant to all cancers, so I included this short essay on it.

Oral Cancer Doesn't Always Present with Visible Clinical Lesions or Pain
It may just look like a simple periapical lesion on one tooth that a dentist treated with root canal therapy and then another and then another.

A patient was referred to our clinic for evaluation and treatment of "apical abscesses" that were unresponsive to endodontic therapy. I was asked to retreat or perform an apicoectomy. This was a 44-year-old Caucasian female with no cc of pain or swelling, and she was told by her dentist to come to this appointment to fix the roots. Her PMH was noncontributory, and she had no medical contraindications to dental treatment. HPI revealed that over the past year and a half, she had seen her dentist for routine dental prophylaxis, and her radiographs.revealed a single loculated radiolucency above the apex of her maxillary central incisors that was treated by her dentist with endodontic therapy and composite resins. A review of her dental records indicated the patient was asymptotic with vital teeth, no mobility, no periodontal probing depths greater than 3mm, and no carious lesions of the teeth throughout her entire dentition. Treatment of maxillary central incisors was initiated due to the radiographic findings.

Exam revealed all CN's II-XII were intact, pt was sans adenopathy, dysphagia, trismus and was afebrile. Her EOMI was intact, and her pupils were PERRLA. She presented with no clinical signs or symptoms of systemic odontogenic infection. Intraoral examination revealed the same as her dental records with minimal plaque score, no errhythema at the free gingival margins, and the only abnormality was a noted slight expansion of the facial cortical plate that was depressible slightly. It was determined to do an FNA and culture to determine the cause of this persistent lesion. The final diagnosis was Ameloblastic Carcinoma. The treatment was anterior maxillectomy, at the university hospital, after healing an obturator and maxillary removable partial denture was fabricated in our clinic.

The takeaway here is that if you have any symptoms and they don't go away or are not relieved by initial treatments, get a second opinion, just like my journey to the diagnosis of ALS.

The patient has been cancer-free as of five year follow up.

PS: Moral of the story—Not every periapical lucency is an endo lesion. The clinical exam should give rise to suspicion. A lesson from my father was while common things occur commonly, and even if it walks like a duck and quacks like a duck, every once in a while, we get a zebra!

CHAPTER 24

RANDOM THOUGHTS—

JUDGING OTHERS' WORK

There's an adage, "Medical school graduates colleagues. Dental school graduates competition."

I *never* judge single restorations or results when looking at others' clinical work. I was not in the operatory. I didn't see the patient, who may have a neurological issue, personality disorder, or is just plain mean and difficult.

That said, I have been asked to review specific cases, and there are some licensed practitioners that require retraining or disciplinary actions. Those here are making an effort to improve, so kudos for all who contribute and attempt to improve.

My advice is to never talk bad about another dentist or other healthcare professional unless it is in a court case. It will always come full circle.

This was a topic over lunch, and we talked about the circuitous route my ALS diagnosis took. One doctor said they took too long and that there should be a head on the proverbial platter, and it reminded me of this line of thought.

I was there and couldn't think of a cleaner, straighter line to the truth. Sometimes, it just takes a tincture of time.

CHAPTER 25

RANDOM THOUGHTS—THERE ARE MULTIPLE

OPTIONS IN HEALTHCARE

A LS care shouldn't be my way or the highway. I wrote this for dentists, but it really is true for those of us dealing with ALS. Dentistry is like medicine, not religion, where there is one only perfect way to get to heaven. I can and have treated hemorrhoids with ointments (nitroglycerin and antibiotics), whereas a surgeon would band or do a Doppler guided rectal arterectomy, one of the most painful operations there is. There is more than one way to fix or replace a tooth.

Quality. . . Depending on what you see in training, the clinical cut off for treatments by clinicians runs the gamut from substandard to textbook examples of excellence. My pearl is to train with the best look at Pankey, go to Christianson, join the AGD, pursue a Fellowship, and then Mastership, then take the board certification in general dentistry.

For the past thirty-three years, I've had several instances where I could justify a cast restoration on a particular tooth, but the patient had no resources for expensive dental restoration. I have used both amalgam and composite resins to build up severely damaged teeth and followed them for decades, now. Circumstances change, and I and my associate dentists routinely see these same patients and, when necessary, we restore these same teeth with crowns

Long story short, these build-ups have lasted as long as crowns.

Besides the prescription meds approved for ALS, none of which offer a cure, there are many ways to increase overall health to buy time until a real cure is available.

CHAPTER 26

RANDOM THOUGHTS—MEDICAL EMERGENCIES

IN DENTAL PRACTICE

I wrote this after treating a closed head injury in the median of a busy Interstate Highway 2018.

I handled a medical emergency involving an unconscious patient while onboard a nonstop flight to Florida from St. Louis in June of 2016. In October 1995, I decompressed a pneumothorax on a street curb after a man suffered a gunshot wound to the chest.

While in my dental residency and medical school, I ran codes and was a certified instructor in Advanced Cardiac Life Support and as a provider in Advanced Trauma Life Support. The best way to prevent emergencies is to prevent them, but the best way to handle them is to train.

Medical emergencies occur everywhere. If you care for an ALS patient, be prepared as much as you can.

How many of you are prepared today to treat a medical emergency in your office, or even in the street?

This event occurred on 6 May 2018, sixty miles south of Memphis around 1:00 p.m.

Immediately after dental school, I trained and certified in Advanced Trauma Life Support (ATLS) and Advanced Cardiac Life Support (ACLS) as preparation for medical emergencies as a United States Navy officer.

During my career, I have treated gunshot wounds in the middle of the street in St. Louis. I have treated medical emergencies like an unconscious passenger aboard commercial airlines as well as a myriad of medical emergencies in the hospital and the dental clinics.

Yesterday, while riding my motorcycle back to St. Louis from an annual crawfish eating binge and party in Lafayette, La., I rode up to a horrific motorcycle accident scene. I was the only doctor on the scene for ten minutes. During that time, we called 911 and then assessed the injured victim. The victim was in critical condition with multiple fractures including skull, arm, ribs, internal.

My wife took this shot. I am wearing a yellow shirt under a motorcycle club vest that has my club's blue patch on the back.

Are you ready? You never know when Miss. or Mrs. or Mr. X walks in so they can have their heart attack . . . I mean their crown cemented.

CHAPTER 27

RANDOM THOUGHTS—PREVENTION

THROUGH EXERCISE

This is another *Dental Clinical Pearls* post I made a few years into my diagnosis of ALS.

Thoughts on Preventive Medicine

If you have ALS, you can benefit from exercise.

Archives of Internal Medicine, Dec, '09 article on sedentary elderly individuals reports older, seasoned citizens benefit from exercise. Use it or lose it. The article showed increased longevity, decreased depression, and increased mental function. As I said in the discussion I had yesterday with a patient, "What are you waiting for? The first potentially fatal heart attack?" It is never too late to try.

Thought for today: Bainbridge reflex! Exercise your legs. Your legs are your second heart. The stronger your legs, the stronger your heart beats. Walk, then run, then lift yourself to a healthier you.

Maintaining your own health will help you not only practice but will increase the quality of your entire life. The Pearl here is to do absolutely everything you know to maintain your health. Even when physicians offer no hope, educate yourself. You are your best health advocate.

While waiting for discharge from the hospital and reflecting on the absolutely stellar care I received from my surgeon and internist to the hospitalist and the best nurses since Florence Nightingale, I realized Barnes Hospital West made the best of a truly miserable situation, and I am happily thankful.

I much prefer providing healthcare than receiving it. I also understand just how blessed I am to have an understanding of what is happening or what is about to happen, compared to the general population.

Many medical procedures, just like police work, when witnessed by the uninitiated can at first glance appear brutal and painfully unnecessary. Professionals, through training and education, understand the subtle nuances of the hows and especially the whys of doing seemingly invasive actions to another human's body that are designed through science and delivered through artistic interpretation.

I have spent thirty-three years in practice and continued learning, and nothing prepares one for a seemingly hopeless diagnosis, especially when I practiced what I preached. I worked out diligently for my entire adult life (martial arts, CrossFit training under professional tutelage, and prepping for emergent situations as a police officer/dentist/physician). I ate right following what real scientific nutritional journals reported and published clean work. . . think DASH diet on steroids.

The doctors at Washington University and again at St. Louis University told me I have ALS and there is no treatment available (there are a couple of medications that may extend one's life a few months, and the new Radicava that hit the arsenal after the famed Ice Bucket Challenge). I infused this one for about a year. I tried it, after being advised to get my affairs in order as the usual course is two to five years to death. I stopped receiving it in December of 2018.

To all my dental colleagues, I'd like to say that your health is your greatest asset. Without it, a billion dollars won't buy you any more time—time to practice, time for family, time to play and enjoy the fruits of all your arduous work. I have lectured about lifestyle changes necessary to maintain your health, as I believe it is exceedingly difficult to "sell" healthcare when the provider appears to be the opposite of what we are selling.

When 70 percent of healthcare dollars are spent on preventable diseases, it proves we don't have a healthcare crisis in America, we have a health crisis in America. When half of the prescription drugs are written to control the toxic side effects (anti-hypertension meds can slow metabolism, thereby increasing weight; antibiotics, even a single course, can alter gut flora to a point where short-chain fatty acid metabolism is interrupted and a patient's cognitive function is altered; almost any drug with anti as a precursor causes xerostomia and we all know its effects on dentition) of the first half of medications patients are currently taking, and it can be shown in our literature that we could eliminate most of these meds through lifestyle changes. I personally believe it should be our duty to teach our patients how to prevent dental disease and its intimate relationship with a myriad of seemingly unrelated medical conditions. Teaching also means being healthy role models whom our patients seek to emulate.

So, after dealing with ALS symptoms since 1996 and eventually accepting this diagnosis, I chose to do everything necessary to stay on two feet and avoid assuming room temperature. Now, hopefully, sharing a few tips may prolong the time others can enjoy living through increased quality and longevity.

Avoiding obesity is as critical as breathing. An unintended consequence as the American public has gotten sicker over the past several decades is a widening of many of the lab values that are considered normal. You don't want to be in the highs or the lows of normal. Take testosterone as an example or total cholesterol as another. Testosterone was once considered low at 500, and now low normal is 300. Cholesterol just below 200 is now high normal, when 150 and below were once a marker for concern.

We as a profession are sedentary, and what was once considered just aging (such as the expansion of our waistlines) is now recognized as pathology. Just like older medical texts used to say the periodontal disease was a normal part of aging, we now recognize it is usual but hardly normal.

Reducing weight and maintaining a healthy weight is essential in reducing one's chances of developing hypertension, diabetes, arteriosclerosis.

A good read for those inclined to get or stay healthy is Michael Greger's book, *How Not to Die.*

CHAPTER 28

RANDOM THOUGHTS—DENTISTRY, ULCERS, AND ALS

I posted this on *Dental Clinical Pearls.*

Decreasing VDO, Lemons and REFLUX, and Limes Oh My
Patients with ALS present with GI symptoms like constipation, which causes painful abdominal swelling bloating and inability to be comfortable in a dental chair. These patients also present with burning and belching from acid in the stomach and other contents coming back up into the mouth. The treatment of this burning and belching can increase the patient's quality of life.

An earlier post got me to thinking about GERD, what we know about it now, how the treatment for this has changed, and why we as dentists should be advocates for our patients and communicate with their primary care physicians when we see the oral effects of this dangerous systemic condition.

If your patients have a chief complaint of belching or burning in their stomach or chest, particularly when the stomach is empty, they probably have either an infection, a tumor, or a condition called GERD (reflux or regurgitation). Infection with bacteria such as *helicobacter pylori* is by far the most common cause (over 90 percent).

Their primary care doctor will probably order a series of laboratory tests and an upper GI series X-ray to rule out a tumor, because we have to rule out zebras for legal reasons, especially when it is proven that over 90 percent of the time, it will not be a diagnosis of any tumor. The blood test for a bacteria called *Helicobacter pylori* should be performed, and the patients should be treated with antibiotics even if the blood test is negative, because there are at least twenty-three other species of bacteria that this test does not detect. Unfortunately, we can be blinded by laboratory science and not see the forest for the trees. Just because a patient is negative for *H pylori*, many docs will not treat their patients with antibiotics. Like HPV and cervical cancer, *H pylori* and the other twenty-three bacteria have been implicated in the development of stomach tumors and cancer. A gastroenterologist will want to perform an endoscopy (putting a tube down through the mouth and into your stomach), often with nebulous results. There are false negatives to this technique, and the biopsy that he will perform can miss not only ulcers but also miss the cultures for *H pylori* (eleven).

When the test for *H pylori* is negative, many primary care physicians will treat for the infection since the literature specifically shows that the other species are not found on routine blood tests. They require PCR and other more expensive tests not covered by insurance or not available in small communities. Many other doctors fall back on the laboratory tests and do not treat. They will diagnosis the patient with GERD and prescribe treatments including a bland diet and acid-blocking drugs. It is the treatment of the symptoms and not the cause that leads to further morbidity, as mentioned earlier these patients with chronic uncleared infection can develop cancers, just like chronic infections with HBV, EBV, HPV. The course of antibiotics may offer a cure for not only the infection and symptoms but also prevent future cancer. Again. journal articles have been published that show at least twenty-four biochemically and morphologically discreet species that can produce these symptoms, yet no test is available for all.

Today, unfortunately, many doctors are still prescribing bland diets and stress reduction while ignoring the work of one of the attending physicians at my alma mater, UVA School of Medicine (GO CAVS!), Dr. Barry Marshall. Dr. Marshall proved ulcers, reflux, hiatal hernia, and GERD were caused by infection. His work earned him the Nobel Prize. To this day, many doctors here in the USA will not let progress get in the way of traditional treatment. Since his original publication, *Helicobacter* has also been associated with several other systemic conditions, including heart attack, peripheral vascular disease, liver conditions, skin eruptions, etc.

D. D. Jines, DMD, MD

Literature backing up the use of antibiotics for the treatment of ulcers:

1. J. G. Kusters, E. J. Kuipers. Non-pylori Helicobacter infections in humans. European Journal of Gastroenterology & Hepatology. 10: 3 (MAR 1998):239–241.
2. J. C. Debongnie, M. Donnay, J. Mairesse, V. Lamy, X. Dekoninck, B. Ramdani. Gastric ulcers and Helicobacter heilmannii. European Journal of Gastroenterology & Hepatology. 10: 3 (MAR 1998):251–254.
3. MA Stone, DB Barnett, JF Mayberry. Lack of correlation between self-reported symptoms of dyspepsia and infection with Helicobacter pylori, in a general population sample. European Journal of Gastroenterology & Hepatology. 10: 4 (1998):301–304.
4. M. Stolte, G. Kroher, A. Meining, A. Morgner, E. Bayerdorffer, B. Bethke. A comparison of Helicobacter pylori and H-heilmannii gastritis-A matched control study involving

404 patients. Scandinavian Journal of Gastroenterology 32:1(JAN 1997):28–33.

5. M. J. Blaser. Heterogeneity of Helicobacter pylori. European Journal of Gastroenterology & Hepatology. 9:Suppl.1 (APR 1997)S3–S6.
6. C. Seidl, V. Grouls, H. J. Schalk. Bulboduodenitis associated with Helicobacter heilmannii (formerly Gastrospirillum hominis) infection. A rare cause of duodenal ulcer. Leber Magen Darm 27: 3 (MAY 1997):156–159.
7. H. Yoshida, K. Hirota, Y. Shiratori, T. Nihei, S. Amano, A. Yoshida, O. Kawamata, M. Omata. Use of a gastric juice-based PCR assay to detect Helicobacter pylori infection in culture-negative patients. Microbiology 36:1(JAN1998):317–320.
8. J. Fox. Helicobacters: the next generation. Baillieres Clinical Infectious Diseases 4: 3(NOV 1997):449–471.
9. A. Meining, G. Kroher, M. Stolte. Animal reservoirs in the transmission of Helicobacter heilmannii—Results of a questionnaire-based study. Scandinavian Journal of Gastroenterology 33: 8(AUG 1998):795–798. dogs, chickens cats, cattle, or pigs reservoirs in the transmission of H. heilmannii. J Fox. Helicobacters: the next generation. Baillieres Clinical Infectious Diseases 4: 3(NOV 1997):449–471. dogs, cats, ferrets, pigs, monkeys and cheetahs, other mammals, and birds. mice H. canis, H. rappini and H. pullorum isol To date, there are at least 19 formally named species of the new genus, Helicobacter.
10. Monkeys have so many different bacteria in their stomachs that nobody can tell what belongs there or is causing stomach symptoms. The bacteria that were found were susceptible to the following antibiotics: amikacin, ciprofloxacin, gentamicin, cefoperazone, tobramycin, imipenem, and trimethoprim/ sulfamethoxazole. S. S. Khanolkar Gaitonde, G. K. Reubish, C. K. Lee, C. T. K. H. Stadtlander. Isolation

of bacteria other than Helicobacter pylori from stomachs of squirrel monkeys (Saimiri spp.) with gastritis. Digestive Diseases and Sciences, 2000, Vol 45, Iss 2, pp 272–280.

11. R. Colin, P. Czernichow, V. Baty, I. Touze, F. Brazier, J. F. Bretagne, I. Berkelmans, P. Barthelemy, J. Hemet. Low sensitivity of invasive tests for the detection of Helicobacter pylori infection in patients with bleeding ulcers. Gastroenterologie Clinique et Biologique, 2000, Vol 24, Iss 1, pp 31–35.

12. Helicobacter mesocricetorum sp nov., a novel helicobacter isolated from the feces of Syrian hamsters. Journal of Clinical Microbiology, 2000, Vol 38, Iss 5, pp 1811–1817.

13. K. Mention, L. Michaud, D. Guimber, E. M. DeLasalle, P. Vincent, D. Turck, F. Gottrand. Characteristics and prevalence of Helicobacter heilmannii infection in children undergoing upper gastrointestinal endoscopy. Journal of Pediatric Gastroenterology and Nutrition, 1999, Vol 29, Iss 5, pp 533–539.

14. P. Vandamme, C. S. Harrington, K. Jalava, S. L. W. On. Misidentifying helicobacters: the Helicobacter cinaedi example. Journal of Clinical Microbiology, 2000, Vol 38, Iss 6, pp 2261–2266.

15. P. Ferenci. The importance of Helicobacter - Also beyond the stomach. Acta Medica Austriaca, 2000, Vol 27, Iss 4, pp 109–111.

16. The non-H pylori helicobacters: their expanding role in gastrointestinal and systemic diseases. Gut, 2002, Vol 50, Iss 2, pp 273–283. J. G. Fox. MIT, Div Comparat Med, 77 Massachusetts Ave, Bldg 16, Room 825C, Cambridge, MA 02139 USA

17. Highly effective second-line anti-Helicobacter pylori therapy in patients with previously failed metronidazole-based therapy. Scandinavian Journal of Gastroenterology 32:12(Dec 1997):1209–1214.

18. N. A. Alsomal, K. E. Coley, P. C. Molan, B. M. Hancock. Role of Helicobacter Pylori Serology in Evaluating Treatment Success. Digestive Diseases and Sciences 1993 (Dec);38(12): 2262–2266.

19. W. M. Wang, C. Y. Chen, C. M. Jan, L. T. Chen, D. S. Perng, S. R. Lin, C. S. Liu. Long term follow up and serological study after triple therapy of Helicobacter pylori-associated duodenal ulcer. American Journal of Gastroenterology 89: 10(OCT 1994):1793–1796.

20. M. A. Mendall, R. P. Jazrawi, J. M. Marrero, N. Molineaux, J. Levi, J. D. Maxwell, T.C. Northfield. Serology for Helicobacter pylori compared with symptom question-naires in screening before direct access endoscopy. Gut 36:3 (MAR 1995):330–333.

21. Z. Maratka. Endoscopic diagnosis of gastritis: Pros and Cons. Journal of Clinical Gastroenterology 20:2(MAR 1995):92–93. The endoscopic characteristics of inflamma-tion in the stomach, in contrast to those of the esophagus and colon, are inconspicuous or lacking, "Endoscopic gastri-tis" does not correlate sufficiently with "histologic gastritis" and the term "gastritis" is to be limited to cases confirmed histologically.

22. C. A. Fallone, G. E. Wild, C. A. Goresky, A. N. Barkun. Evaluation of IgA and IgG serology for the detection of Helicobacter pylori infection. Canadian Journal of Gastroenterology 9: 2(MAR-APR 1995):105–111.

23. T. U. Kosunen. Antibody titres in Helicobacter pylori infection: Implications in the follow-up of antimicro-bial therapy. Annals of Medicine 27: 5 (OCT 1995):605–607. Success in eradication is reflected in 40-50 percent decrease of antibody titres within five to six months. The decrease continues and most patients have normal titres within two years.

24. R. J. F. Laheij, J. B. M. J. Jansen, E. H. Vandelisdonk, A. L. M. Verbeek. Review article: Symptom improvement through eradication of Helicobacter pylori in patients with non-ulcer dyspepsia. Alimentary Pharmacology & Therapeutics 10: 6(DEC 1996):843–850. 8) M. Feldman, B. Cryer, E. Lee, W. L. Peterson. Role of seroconversion in confirming cure of Helicobacter pylori infection. JAMA, 280:4(JUL 22 1998):363–365

25. M. A. Asante, M. Mendall, P. Patel, L. Ballam, T. C. Northfield. A randomized trial of endoscopy vs no endoscopy in the management of seronegative Helicobacter pylori dyspepsia. European Journal of Gastroenterology & Hepatology. 10: 12 (DEC 1998):983–989.

26. McCarthy, C, et al. Digestive Diseases and Sciences 1995;40:114–119.

27. Kuipers E. J., at al. Atrophic gastritis and helicobacter pylori infection in patients with reflux esophagitis treated with omeperazole or fundoplication. NEJM, 1996(April 18);334(16):1018–1022.

28. C. Omorain, M. Buckley. Helicobacter pylori and dyspepsia. Scandinavian Journal of Gastroenterology. 31: Suppl. 214 (1996):28–30. 6778 4/7/96

29. B. S. Sheu, C. Y. Lin, Z. X. Lin, S. C. Shiesh, H. B. Yang, C. Y. Chen. Long-term outcome of triple therapy in Helicobacter pylori-related nonulcer dyspepsia: A prospective controlled assessment. American Journal of Gastroenterology 91: 3 (MAR 1996):441–447. Compared with control therapy at 1 yr, triple therapy showed greater symptomatic, serological, and histological improvements. Therefore, triple therapy is beneficial to symptomatic HP-related NUD.

30. S. Khulusi, S. Badve, P. Patel, R. Lloyd, J. M. Marrero, C. Finlayson, M. A. Mendall, T. C. Northfield. Pathogenesis of gastric metaplasia of the human duodenum: Role

of Helicobacter pylori, gastric acid, and ulceration. Gastroenterology 110: 2 (FEB 1996):452–458. This study shows that the extent of duodenal GM is unrelated to the presence or absence of ulceration but is partly due to H. pylori and partly due to acid.

31. Annals of Internal Medicine August 15, 1995;123:260–268.

32. B. J. Marshall. Managing acid peptic disease in the Helicobacter pylori era. Journal of Clinical Gastroenterology 21: Suppl. 1(1995):S155–S159. The advent of new diagnostic and therapeutic modalities for Helicobacter pylori allows any physician to offer curative antibiotic regimens to patients with peptic ulcer disease and gastritis. In the new strategy, patients with dyspepsia are investigated with serology to detect those with H. pylori and potentially curable peptic ulcers. Only those who are H. pylori-negative undergo endoscopy.

33. A. F. Cutler, V. M. Prasad. Long-term follow-up of Helicobacter pylori serology after successful eradication. American Journal of Gastroenterology 91: 1 (JAN 1996):85–88. A 20 percent decline in IgG concentration has an overall sensitivity of 93 percent for determining H. pylori eradication twelve to twenty-one months after H. pylori treatment.

34. M. Buckley, C. Omorain. Prevalence of Helicobacter pylori in non-ulcer dyspepsia. Alimentary Pharmacology & Therapeutics 9: Suppl. 2(1995):53–58.

35. A. F. Cutler, V. M. Prasad. Long-term follow-up of Helicobacter pylori serology after successful eradication. American Journal of Gastroenterology 91: 1 (JAN 1996):85–88. A 20 percent decline in IgG concentration has an overall sensitivity of 93 percent for determining H. pylori eradication twelve to twenty-one months after H. pylori treatment.

36. P. A. Testoni, E. Colombo, L. Cattani, M. Longhi, F. Bagnolo, F. Lella, M. Buizza, R. Scelsi. Helicobacter pylori serology

in chronic gastritis with antral atrophy and negative histology for Helicobacter-like organisms. Journal of Clinical Gastroenterology 22: 3 (APR 1996):182–185.

37. M. Plebani, D. Basso, M. Cassaro, L. Brigato, M. Scrigner, A. Toma, F. Dimario, M. Rugge. Helicobacter pylori serology in patients with chronic gastritis. American Journal of Gastroenterology 91: 5 (MAY 1996):954–958. Helicobacter pylori (Hp) serum IgG and Pepsinogen most accurately indicated Hp infection, and their product mag he proposed as an aid in diagnosing Hp infection in dyspeptic patients.

38. H. Kawaguchi, K. Haruma, K. Komoto, M. Yoshihara, K. Sumii, G. Kajiyama. Helicobacter pylori infection is the major risk factor for atrophic gastritis. American Journal of Gastroenterology 91: 5 (MAY 1996):959–962. 14) J. Labenz, T. Rokkas. Helicobacter pylori and dyspepsia. Current Opinion in Gastroenterology 13: Suppl. 1(1997): A. Heaney, J. S. A. Collins, R. G. P. Watson, R. J. McFarland, K. B. Bamford, T. C. K. Tham. A prospective randomised trial of a "test and treat" policy versus endoscopy based management in young Helicobacter pylori positive patients with ulcer-like dyspepsia, referred to a hospital clinic. Gut, 1999, Vol 45, Iss 2, pp 186–190.

39. S. Tefera, J. G. Hatlebakk, A. Berstad. The effect of Helicobacter pylori eradication on gastro-oesophageal reflux. Alimentary Pharmacology & Therapeutics, 1999, Vol 13, Iss 7, pp 915–920. Twelve weeks after H. Pylori eradication there was no consistent change in gastro-oesophageal acid reflux in patients with mild or moderate reflux oesophagitis.

40. F. T. M. Peters, E. J. Kuipers, S. Ganesh, W. J. Sluiter, E. C. KlinkenbergKnol, C. B. H. W. Lamers, J. H. Kleibeuker. The influence of Helicobacter pylori on oesophageal

acid exposure in GERD during acid-suppressive therapy. Alimentary Pharmacology & Therapeutics, 1999, Vol 13, Iss 7, pp 921–926.

41. M. Stolte, G. Kroher, A. Meining, A. Morgner, E. Bayerdorffer, B. Bethke. A comparison of Helicobacter pylori and H-heilmannii gastritis-A matched control study involving 404 patients. Scandinavian Journal of Gastroenterology 32:1 (JAN 1997):28–33.

42. C. Dieterich, P. Wiesel, R. Neiger, A. Blum, I. Corthesytheulaz. Presence of multiple "Helicobacter heilmannii" strains in an individual suffering from ulcers and in his two cats. Journal of Clinical Microbiology 36: 5 (MAY 1998): 1366–1370.

43. M. Giladi, A. Lembo, B. L. Johnson. Postural epigastric pain: A unique symptom of primary cytomegalovirus gastritis? Infection 26: 4 (JUL–AUG 1998):234–235.

44. R. J. Owen. Helicobacter - species classification and identification. British Medical Bulletin 54: 1 (1998):17–30.

45. N. Kitamoto, H. Nakamoto, A. Katai, N. Takahara, H. Nakata, H. Tamaki, T. Tanaka. Heterogeneity of protein profiles of Helicobacter pylori isolated from individual patients. Helicobacter 3: 3 (SEP 1998):152–162.

46. C. F. Li, T. Z. Ha, D. A. Ferguson, D. S. Chi, R. G. Zhao, N. R. Patel, G. Krishnaswamy, E. Thomas. A newly developed PCR assay of H-pylori in gastric biopsy, saliva, and feces: Evidence of high prevalence of H-pylori in saliva supports oral transmission. Digestive Diseases and Sciences 41: 11 (NOV 1996):2142–2149.

47. K. Schutze, E. Hentschel, B. Dragosics, A. M. Hirschl. Helicobacter pylori reinfection with identical organisms: Transmission by the patients' spouses. Gut 36: 6 (JUN 1995):831–833.

48. Infection and Immunity 1994;62:2367–74.

49. K. Shankaran, H. G. Desai. Helicobacter pylori in dental plaque. Journal of Clinical Gastroenterology 21:2(SEP 1995):82–84.
50. F. Parente, G. Maconi, O. Sangaletti, M. Minguzzi, L. Vago, E. Rossi, G. B. Porro. Prevalence of Helicobacter pylori infection and related gastroduodenal lesions in spouses of Helicobacter pylori-positive patients with duodenal ulcer. Gut 39: 5 (NOV 1996):629–633.
51. S. D. Georgopoulos, A. F. Mentis, C. A. Spiliadis, L. S. Tzouvelekis, E. Tzelepi, A. Moshopoulos, N. Skandalis. Helicobacter pylori infection in spouses of patients with duodenal ulcers and comparison of ribosomal RNA gene patterns. Gut 39: 5 (NOV 1996):634–638.
52. C. Dieterich, P. Wiesel, R. Neiger, A. Blum, I. Corthesytheulaz. Presence of multiple "Helicobacter heilmannii" strains in an individual suffering from ulcers and in his two cats. Journal of Clinical Microbiology 36: 5 (MAY 1998):1366–1370.
53. Meining, G. Kroher, M. Stolte. Animal reservoirs in the transmission of Helicobacter heilmannii - Results of a questionnaire-based study. Scandinavian Journal of Gastroenterology 33: 8(AUG 1998):795–798.
54. N. Chiba, A. B. R. Thomson, P. Sinclair. From bench to bedside to bug: An update of clinically relevant advances in the care of persons with Helicobacter pylori-associated diseases. Canadian Journal of Gastroenterology, 2000, Vol 14, Iss 3, pp 188–198.
55. NEJM, July 25, 1996 R. Barretozuniga, M. Maruyama, Y. Kato, K. Aizu, H. Ohta, T. Takekoshi, S. F. Bernal. Significance of Helicobacter pylori infection as a risk factor in gastric cancer: Serological and histological studies. Journal of Gastroenterology 32: 3 (JUN 1997):289–294.
56. J. H. Siman, A. Forsgren, G. Berglund, C. H. Floren. Association between Helicobacter pylori and gastric

carcinoma in the city of Malmo, Sweden-A prospective study. Scandinavian Journal of Gastroenterology 32: 12(DEC 1997):1215–1221.

57. E. Ierardi, R. Francavilla, C. Panella. Effect of Helicobacter pylori eradication on intestinal metaplasia and gastric epithelium proliferation. Italian Journal of Gastroenterology and Hepatology. 29: 5 (OCT 1997):470–475.

58. S. Tsuji, M. Tsujii, W. H. Sun, E. S. Gunawan, H. Murata, S. Kawano, M. Hori. Helicobacter pylori and gastric carcinogenesis. Journal of Clinical Gastroenterology. 25: Suppl. 1(1997): S186–S197.

59. R. Cheli, M. Crespi, G. Testino, F. Citarda. Gastric cancer and Helicobacter pylori: Biologic and epidemiologic inconsistencies. Journal of Clinical Gastroenterology 26: 1 (JAN 1998):3–6.

60. V. Pasceri, G. Cammarota, G. Patti, L. Cuoco, A. Gasbarrini, R. L. Grillo, G. Fedeli, G. Gasbarrini, A. Maseri. Association of virulent Helicobacter pylori strains with ischemic heart disease. Circulation 97: 17 (MAY 5 1998):1675–1679.48–51. J. Danesh. Helicobacter pylori infection and gastric cancer: systemic review of the epidemiological studies.Alimentary Pharmacology & Therapeutics, 1999, Vol 13, Iss 7, pp 851–856.

61. K. Haruma, K. Komoto, T. Kamada, M. Ito, Y. Kitadai, M. Yoshihara, K. Sumii, G. Kajiyama. Helicobacter pylori infection is a major risk factor for gastric carcinoma in young patients. Scandinavian Journal of Gastroenterology, 2000, Vol 35, Iss 3, pp 255–259.

62. J. W. Konturek, A. Dembinski, S. J. Konturek, J. Stachura, W. Domschke. Infection of Helicobacter pylori in gastric adaptation to continued administration of aspirin in humans. Gastroenterology 114: 2 (FEB 1998):245–255.

63. R. I. Russell. Helicobacter pylori eradication may reduce the risk of gastroduodenal lesions in chronic NSAID users. Italian Journal of Gastroenterology and Hepatology. 29: 5 (OCT 1997):465–469.

64. C. Y. Wu, S. K. Poon, G. H. Chen. Is Helicobacter pylori a risk factor for NSAID- associated gastric ulcer bleeding? A sex- and age-matched case-control study. Advances in Therapy 15: 2 (MAR-APR 1998):85–91.

65. M. Stolte, G. Kroher, A. Meining, A. Morgner, E. Bayerdorffer, B. Bethke. A comparison of Helicobacter pylori and H-heilmannii gastritis-A matched control study involving 404 patients. Scandinavian Journal of Gastroenterology 32:1(JAN 1997):28–33.

66. M. J. Blaser. Hetero-geneity of Helicobacter pylori. European Journal of Gastroenterology & Hepatology. 9: Suppl.1 (APR 1997)S3–S6.

67. C. Seidl, V. Grouls, H. J. Schalk. Bulboduodenitis associated with Helicobacter heilmannii (formerly Gastrospirillum hominis) infection. A rare cause of duodenal ulcer. Leber Magen Darm 27: 3 (MAY 1997):156–159.

68. H. Yoshida, K. Hirota, Y. Shiratori, T. Nihei, S. Amano, A. Yoshida, O. Kawamata, M. Omata. Use of a gastric juice-based PCR assay to detect Helicobacter pylori infection in culture-negative patients. Microbiology 36:1(JAN1998):317–320.

69. D. Scott, D. Weeks, K. Melchers, G. Sachs. The life and death of Helicobacter pylori. Gut 43: Suppl. 1 (JUL 1998):S56–S60. In the absence of division, antibiotics such as clarithromycin and amoxicillin are ineffective. Proton pump inhibitors, by elevating gastric pH, would increase the population of dividing organisms and hence synergize with these antibiotics.

CHAPTER 29

RANDOM THOUGHTS—DENTISTRY AND

HYPERTENSION

I posted this on the *Dental Clinical Pearls* website.

Dentistry and A Professional Risk Factor—Hypertension
Our work is stressful and demands much of us physically. Not that dental work requires the physical activity of a ditch-digging laborer but just the opposite. We are sedentary and sit in posture torturing positions guaranteed to get you looking down in the mouth over time.

During my medical training, I became aware of an unfortunate and seemingly, or should I say hopefully, an unintended consequence of unhealthy lifestyles: the poly-pharmacy merry-go-round. Today, approximately half the medications prescribed are to manage the side effects of medications patients already take. Now, combine that with the fact that 70percent of our healthcare dollars are spent on conditions that a healthy lifestyle could prevent, and you come to the realization that I have posted here before: We don't have a healthcare crisis in America. We have a health crisis.

Many of you will develop hypertension, and your primary care physician will prescribe anti-hypertension medication to treat you. Dentists out there, please take note that the most effective anti-hypertension meds work in the range of 30–40 percent of the time at getting your BP down to safe levels. Every hypertension medication has a negative side effect. Some will slow your metabolism and you will gain weight, which in turn will raise your blood pressure . . . but that is okay because I have another medication for that. See how the merry-go-round works? Some meds will cause fluid retention, but then again, there's a medicine we have for that, and so on and so forth.

Back in 2000, a paper was published after researchers at Harvard, Duke, and Johns Hopkins showed a diet now called DASH (Dietary Approaches to Stop Hypertension) to control blood pressure better than meds. This work has since been shown to control hypertension and control adult-onset diabetes 88 percent of the time within just two weeks, and it works before the patients even lose much weight. This diet can help patients lose weight and reverse adult-onset diabetes as well as control hypertension.

I regularly tell all my patients with hypertension and diabetes about this diet. My question to all you dentists taking hypertension meds is, "Did your physician tell you about this diet, and if not, why?"

1. P. R. Conlin, D. Chow, E. R. Miller, L. P. Svetkey, P. H. Lin, D. W. Harsha, T. J. Moore, F. M. Sacks, L. J. Appel. The effect of dietary patterns on blood pressure control in hypertensive patients: Results from the Dietary Approaches to Stop Hypertension (DASH) trial. American Journal of Hypertension, 2000, Vol 13, Iss 9, pp 949–955.
2. L. M. Resnick, S. Oparil, A. Chait, R. B. Haynes, P. KrisEtherton, J. S. Stern, S. Clark, S. Holcomb, D. C. Hatton, J. A. Metz, M. McMahon, F.X. PiSunyer, D. A. McCarron.

Factors affecting blood pressure responses to diet: The vanguard study. American Journal of Hypertension, 2000, Vol 13, Iss 9, pp 956–965.
3. Circulation. September, 2000
4. American Journal of Hypertension, 2001, Vol 14, Iss 6, Part 2, Suppl. S, pp 206S–212S

D. D. Jines, DMD, MD

CHAPTER 30

RANDOM THOUGHTS—HIV/AIDS

P osted this on Clinical Dental Pearls Website

HIV/AIDS in Dentistry Today

Here are three cases of Kaposi's Sarcoma. These are archive images. There are several I have from the earlier days when the life expectancy for individuals diagnosed with AIDS was approximately eighteen to twenty-four months. We have come a very long way since the initial cases were reported back in 1981 or the initial clinical work that led to the reported cases of the most common oral manifestations of HIV/AIDS. I am posting these because I saw an earlier post asking for a differential, but by the time I read the post, there were several great answers.

First, some background on where I am approaching this subject. I graduated dental school (Washington University) in 1985, then completed advance clinical rotations (Great Lakes Naval Dental Clinic and Hospital) and training while in the Navy, before my residency and medical degree (University of Virginia and AISM). Since entering private practice full time, I have served as a clinical instructor of surgery at St. Louis University School of

Medicine, MATEC lecturer on HIV/AIDS as well as Washington University Barnes Hospital AIDS Clinical Trial Unit, and SLU's Vaccine Centers Dental and Oral Medicine consultant. Currently, my clinic has approximately 1,500 HIV patients and about half of our daily fifty to sixty patients are positive.

So, here's the clinical pearl: You are ALL treating a patient who is positive for HIV or Hep C or . . . You should ALL be treating every patient with the same degree of aseptic technique and universal precautions to avoid cross-contamination. In dentistry especially, we have done a great job.

With the advent of aggressive antiretroviral therapies, patients diagnosed with HIV today should live to life expectancy. With proper monitoring and compliance to their medical cocktails, patients can be immune-competent and have undetectable viral loads, thereby making the long list of "The most Common Oral manifestations of HIV/AIDS" almost extinct.

I performed interlesional chemotherapy with Methotrexate and Thalidomide as well as surgical excision of KS lesions like this but fortunately, today, it is almost gone. There are more non-AIDS KS today than those we treated just twenty years ago.

Today, I tell every newly-diagnosed HIV positive patient the history of this condition and that they can look forward to an essentially normal lifestyle with the caveat that they must be better attuned to their healthcare needs and lifestyle habits that can either help or greatly hinder their well-being. We all know that the vast majority of smokers lose their teeth. Smoking destroys a patient's health, including their immune system. The one thing that almost all of my long-term survivors have in common is they are non-smokers. We are dealing with an ever-increasing aging population, and our HIV patients are suffering from the same maladies as everyone who is entering senior status. Yes, these conditions like diabetes, hypertension, arteriosclerosis, cancers are all complicated by their immune status, and we in the field of dentistry can help save lives by eliminating sources of systemic odontogenic infections.

Educating these patients (I have oft said that doctor means teacher) about the hows and whys of dental hygiene can save not only one's dentition but their life. Decreasing chronic bacteremia caused by chronic periodontal disease lowers levels of CRP, thereby lowering the risk of not only heart valve damage and increased risk of stroke and acute coronary events, it also reduces localized reactive arthritis and difficulties in diabetes management . . . Hopefully, you are getting the picture.

Early on, we could culture the cause of PCP (at one time, the leading cause of AIDS deaths) from the mouths of patients before we could culture it from the lungs. Histoplasmosis and CMV, which are endemic, could be found easily as well. Today, when a patient is well-controlled with their meds, it is becoming a rarity once again to see these killers. Oral fungal infections are again a function of decreased vertical dimension or chronic denture wear instead of compromised immune function.

Look at the most common oral manifestations of HIV/AIDS and treatments for didactic exercise and understanding, and you are in the driver's seat for early detection. If a patient is unaware of their status and presents with chronic refractory fungal infections, suspect immune compromise and refer to their primary care physician and ask for testing and diagnosis of the etiology. They will know what to do, for I am there.

Last thought on this is to treat these and all patients to eliminate any source of infection, and you will greatly improve your patients' overall health, and for the most part, make many of the original oral manifestations of HIV/AIDS a distant memory.

D. D. Jines, DMD, MD

CHAPTER 31

RANDOM THOUGHTS—THEY CALL IT PRACTICE

FOR A REASON

The following was a post on my Facebook. It's just a description of my day. ALS was not a conscious thought.

Social Media: Always Posting the Best Cases and Taking an Unusually, Strangely Uncharacteristic Day in Stride

The day before I head off to Canada for annual Motorcycle Club meeting—twelve hours, eight-hundred miles—all I have to do is see my patients, then fuel up and go. What could go wrong? Never ask what could go wrong. It will. It does.

So, today, 8 August 2018. started great. Removed impacted wisdom teeth from my favorite medical student, texted with my globetrotting youngest who is in Munich, and then did the daily rounds with patients and life. By 2:00 p.m., with just a couple of hours to go, I had a patient prove retraction cord with a couple of drops hemodent could make them vomit their Steak and Shake chili cheese fries and coke.

That's okay. We cleaned up and off to the next procedure. Crown delivery. Temp fits die, crown seats perfectly, contacts good, occlusion stellar. Porcelain breaks as I have a patient bite on an orange stick. Mesial buccal cusp tip on PFM fractures, giving the appearance of a class VI amalgam. Rescheduled to just redo crown. Many ways to fix a problem, but I'd rather just get it right the first time or do it over.

The afternoon is shaping up nicely, so let me just deliver another crown, but wait . . . the remaining tooth broke off while removing temporary. Oh, what fresh hell hath . . . emergently temporize so we can now rebuild, reprep, and reimpress.

Oh, well, this next patient coming in has been a patient thirty years and only requires endodontic treatment of number nineteen. Great final fill after obturating the distal canal twice.

Why post this? It's simple. We are responsible for how we react to every situation. We own our actions. We choose happiness or anger. Choose wisely.

Now, let the fun and extended weekend begin.

CHAPTER 32

RANDOM THOUGHTS—POLITICS

My patient asked me what I thought about guns.

Random Thoughts about Self Defense

Does a momma panda bear have a right to defend its den from a poacher or another animal trying to steal or eat its young? Natural Law would say yes. What is different for people?

For a free country to exist, it must have a moral people, and if moral, then must they believe in a god? I think yes. I am not religious and have been trained in science, and the more I've read, the more I understand that there is infinitely more not understood. We are scratching at the surface of knowledge . . . That is for another day.

George Washington once said all government is evil . . . necessary and should be kept small but evil. When people fear a final judgment by their God, they tend to do right. They have a conscience. They believe that even if they are not caught committing a crime, they cannot escape a final judgment from God. In societies that shun the belief in God, they rely on the government to administer punishment sometimes extreme and public. They rely on Big Brother with his all-seeing eye (spy cams, drones) to be the final eyes instead of that internal belief that God is watching so therefore one shouldn't do XYZ. Our Bill of Rights was authored by our forefathers with a belief that our rights come from God and follow natural law. They don't come from the government, and the government cannot take them. Only we can surrender them.

Not being religious doesn't mean I don't believe. I do. I've read several texts and found many to contain truths that can act as instruction manuals. The Christian Bible has been the most instructive to me as it lays out the foundation for democracy, individual salvation and freedom, scientific enlightenment, and a solution to every human malady. From irresponsible personal debt to avarice, greed, the entire list of human weaknesses, gluttony, pride (just remember the Brad Pitt and Morgan Freeman movie *Se7en*), there's a solution contained within the text. Whether reading it as a historical novel with all the sex, violence, and intrigue of any Hollywood tale or as the inspired word of God Almighty, anyone can find the truth within its pages. Modern Christianity runs the gamut of traditional ritualistic Catholicism to an evangelical relationship with our invisible father church services to judgmental authoritarian versions. Luckily for me, I learned a long time ago not to judge. I believe in knowing and having my relationship with my God and leaving it between God and me. Your relationship, or lack thereof, is not my fight. I do call out poor, sick, illegal, stupidly immoral behavior and try to distance myself from it, but I do not judge.

So, what has this got to do with guns? Simple. We have to know our Right to Life doesn't come from a government. With rights come responsibilities, and each individual is responsible for maintaining their own rights.

Cain didn't use a Colt AR-15 to kill Abel. He used an Assault Rock. It was a Hate Crime. I'm being silly here to illustrate a point all rape, murder, etc. are hateful in their very nature. Calling it a HATE crime is great for politicians garnering headlines, but it doesn't help the victim. Calling a rock an assault rock is like calling any weapon an assault weapon. The meaning gets lost in the vagaries of Orwellian doublespeak of our political ruling class.

Any gun is nothing more than a tool. Remember Shane saying that to the little brat in the 1953 Western "Shane." The inanimate gun can be used to destroy or save. It only becomes bad when in the hands of an individual who has evil intent. The only way to stop an evil individual armed with a gun is a good guy armed with a gun. Period.

Utopian pipe dreamers would deny reality and say we can legislate away guns and crime. Everywhere that has been tried, violent crime has increased. It is not the gun, it is the heart of those holding them. 150,000,000 people were murdered by their government in the last century, because absolute power corrupts absolutely. When the government is the only legal holder of firearms, the government has always erased human rights.

But if we could save the life of a child, wouldn't it be worth it? You mean like aborting black babies through the genocidal organization that was created by a bigot? I know that's just a little sidebar, but it does show moral equivalency being stretched to its limit. So, let's save one life.

With every subject in politics, we can breakdown the economics of a subject. What do you mean? Guns are used to kill 30,000 people in the USA every year. This number has remained a constant for a century as the population has more than doubled and the number of guns has quadrupled. Of the 30;000, about 19;000 were suicides. The remaining number 11,000 are then further broken gown by accidents, justifiable homicides, homicides. Three-quarters of all justifiable homicides are by civilians who were protecting themselves during rapes, robberies, kidnappings, etc. A quarter of justifiable homicides are attributed to police. As we look further, the vast majority of murders are committed by a very small subset of career violent criminals and gang members. The overall crime rate in the USA has actually declined over the past four decades. More people are killed by hammer, knives, and ball bats that the dreaded assault rifle.

So, that's the bad what about the good? The FBI compiles crime stats, and their own numbers show civilians use guns to stop crimes two million times yearly. Just the presence of a gun held by a good guy stops millions of crimes without anyone being shot.

Here's an example or analogy that may help. Let's try a Risk vs Benefits analogy.

Each year, 40,000 people die in automobile crashes. We could easily reduce the number by lowering speed limits. No, that won't work people. Break the law and speed, just like criminals illegally possess guns when it is already illegal. We could, however, place governors on every car, truck, and motorcycle, making it impossible to go over 20mph. That one action would render automobiles extremely safe. We accept the number of traffic-related deaths, because we accept the benefits of moving commerce faster, traveling faster to fun destinations, and allowing us to spread out away from the cities. We accept those deaths for risky freedom. Now, 250,000 people die due to medical mistakes yearly. That's nine times more people killed by doctors than guns. Doctors save millions of lives yearly, though. Should we outlaw doctors? 30,000 lives are taken with guns, but millions saved by the same inanimate object.

From a political standpoint, gun control is a racist-in-origin power play that is about the subjugation of one group by another, always couched in flowery rhetorical prose. Hitler said for the first time in history that having gun control would keep our streets safe. The only exception was the six million Jews he slaughtered. Stalin, Mao, Castro, Che, and Pol Pot all agreed. Many in this nation like Bill Ayers who said on record that if they could get into power, they would have to kill off twenty to fifty million Americans to cement power. This is why our founding Fathers wrote a Bill of Rights that required amending the Constitution, which is a difficult process, to guarantee the Second Amendment. The Supreme Court has ruled it is an individual's right. They knew the quill pen would be replaced with modern technology and the First Amendment would be covered just as there has been firearms development. Any country that can build internment camps shouldn't be allowed sole use of firearms. Period.

Even ALS patients deserve the right to life. As an ALS patient, my defensive skill set has been slowly taken from being able to use martial arts to being extremely vulnerable. All men may have been made by God, but Samuel Colt made them equal.

Recently, an able-bodied man attacked a disabled paraplegic man over a disability parking spot. The large, able-bodied man broke the defenseless man's arm.

Wolves will prey on the innocent. In Israel, I have seen armed teachers. This should have happened decades ago. The sheep need to turn the tables on the wicked and condemn those who stab their own in the back. Democrat policies are not kind to Jews. As a charter member of Jews for the Preservation of Firearms Ownership, I have spent almost forty years encouraging the sheep to protect themselves.

The only person safe in a gun-free zone is the killer!

I think I left our conversation at that, telling him I have to go now and fight disease and save lives.

Is Healthcare a Right?

I went to school for fifteen years after high school. I incurred the debt before the rules were retroactively changed to make student debt non-deductible and part of the business expenses. I purchased equipment and a building and insurance, supplies, utilities, taxes, and employed ten people to help me deliver care for my patients. I care for my patients, literally and figuratively, and have provided in excess of a million dollars in charitable care. That's many thousands of dollars yearly over the past thirty-five years here in St. Louis. So, when someone says, "Healthcare is a Right," they are saying the government can come to my house and force me to deliver care. I have a personal responsibility to care, but it is not your right to expect me to render care through the use of force.

Being diagnosed with ALS, a potentially terminal illness (there are a handful of long-term survivors), has actually been positive. We all die; however, many I doubt ever truly live. I don't waste much time now, nor did I before, but now there's a prescient reminder to live in the now and enjoy what I'm doing. Life is too short to get up daily and hate your life's work. I actually loved my work, love my life, and love my staff. So what? ALS is a pre-existing condition that makes me uninsurable. I believe we are all responsible for ourselves, but there are catastrophic conditions and situations that require community help, i.e. government. So, the development of a governmental safety net should be the goal, but never should the government be involved in all our business, including healthcare. Everywhere it has been instituted, including the Scandinavian countries, government universal care is a failure. Even Norway is leaning away from it, now. The proposed spending plans on healthcare by all the presidential candidates on this side of the isle exceeds the total amount of money that the government and every millionaire and billionaire have. Every dime. Yet, it's an ongoing amount of endless spending. The New Green Deal calls for more spending than the Healthcare bill, but as I alluded to earlier, we are already broke.

Some type of middle ground needs to be found for patients dealt a catastrophic blow. I doubt if insurance companies are going to help. Here's an analogy for why pre-existing conditions and insurance are a bad fit. I have a car, a house, and a boat, but I neglected to get insurance. I carelessly forget to check my fireplace and leave while it's still burning. Embers flick out and start a house fire. I lose everything. Then, I call the insurance companies and say I promise to pay them $100 per month, and all the insurance company has to do is pay my $400,000 claim. That kind of business model would and does fail. The companies can spread out the cost of my negligence by charging millions of others, effectively forcing them to pay for me. That's not fair. Charity shouldn't be forced. Even though the same redistributing argument can be made for a governmental safety net in that it is all coming from other people, I believe it would allow greater freedom for all, but hey, I'm just one guy.

Random Thoughts on Being Offended

I was informed that many of my opinions may offend people. If opinions offend anyone, then the offended party is mentally weak. Instead of feeling offended, strengthen your side of the arguments. If swearing hurts you, then again, I cannot imagine living in such a pathetically weak state that mere words can hurt you. My use of colorful profanity is a choice I make without regard to whomever it offends. If you are offended by salty language or my political opinions, you have my sympathy, as I cannot imagine how weak you must be for a word to hurt you, let alone a thought. I actually know that political correctness is a means of silencing free speech and controlling thought. Using a victim status or an offended status is a means to bludgeon anyone else whose speech you disagree with. I don't have the time to waste worrying about feelings. I'm too busy trying to live today, hopefully making a difference to someone else.

CHAPTER 33

RANDOM THOUGHTS—HOLIDAYS, DECEMBER

MOVIE REVIEWS, YEAR IN REVIEW

December is my favorite month of the year.

Random Thoughts—Thursday, 6 December 2018

This date is significant to me. Not only was I about to be taken down by a hidden illness that would end my patient care life, but I was keeping ALS in the backseat right up to that moment.

Thursday clinic time is making me feel like either Charlie Sheen or Donald Trump . . . winning.

I'll admit today that since about 3:00 a.m. when a vivid dream I was having awoken my wife, I've been inside my own head looking through the surreal fog how and why we do things on a daily basis.

Why do some people allow themselves to quit and melt into a puddle of despair? Why do we give ourselves license to lash out at the innocent unaware office worker or service worker or waitress? Why do we become so self-absorbed that I and Me is the only topic on the conversation menu?

We lack empathy and have encouraged an entire generation to become selfishly absorbed enough that the very name of their generation now conjures images of narcissistic willful ignorance and self-centered entitlement.

We, the older generations, are to blame for allowing the soft racism of low expectations to divide us by playing on unearned or undeserved guilt. The lazy, easy way to assuage white collective guilt was to throw money to the less fortunate without regard to the unintended consequences of depriving individuals the rewards of virtue, sacrifice, and true positive self-esteem that comes from hard work and successful outcomes.

We have allowed the failed philosophy of socialism to grow its tentacles into the education system, thereby destroying pride in American Exceptionalism and omitting the true history that adds perspective to the very founding and nature of our republic. Failure and hatred of our society are taught within the walls of academia, along with racial hatred and division, while being couched in comfortable terms like diversity and social justice. Real science is being abandoned in favor of politically driven, "make the facts fit our predrawn conclusions" pseudoscience, i.e. Climate Change. Critical thinking and questioning the narratives of the Big Brother mass media are squelched under the fascistic rule of the political correctness police that demand no debate with their failed philosophy.

Oh, back to empathy . . . Remember, I'm in my head today.

EVERYONE has a struggle. We are not without something that requires an effort that causes stress, etc. It is life. My friend Phil Wenrich, one of the great Motor Officers and riding instructors, served his state for a distinguished career despite living quietly with cystic fibrosis that would eventually rob him of so many friends and also his own lungs. His struggle daily was to breath with 20 percent lung function, not whether his bath water was tepid like mine was today again. We all have struggles.

Putting others first or learning empathy can give us perspective. We had a patient this week with a large parotid cancer, who stoically accepted the news that there's a good statistical probability of the potential loss of a large portion of the lower face, and another patient fretting about a small pimple that was totally benign. I have other friends with diabetes, Alzheimer's, family issues, money problems, debt. Have empathy for one another. We all, every one of us, have a struggle that requires some perspective and empathy and forgiveness and support.

Today, 6 December, is like every other day, except I have to treat a very difficult person who really does not appreciate the extra steps we have taken to ensure the case is successful, painless, artistically cosmetic, and cost-effective (the real issue). Today is going swimmingly well, like every other, even though in the back of my mind, I'm remembering that dream. I still feel like I'm WINNING.

Hey! I got to see a doctor friend as an emergency, and we talked about everyday stuff like any normal day. Remember, it's a normal day. Today, it snowed a bit, just like 6 December 2008. Today, I got a call to schedule a nurse to access my port for Radicava infusions (the fruit of the ALS Ice Bucket Challenge) and that's was a good thing. I had the opportunity to schedule more follow up testing for radiation treatment for prostate cancer to weigh myself. Wow, I'm down 15lbs, and I didn't even have it to lose . . . Today, I had a dream at 3:00 a.m. that was so real, it awakened Darla, and she said I was fighting with someone. In my dream, I was trying to turn Eric around to follow me, but he said he had to go, and I couldn't hold on. It's been ten years to the day since my son Eric died, and just like every other day, life does and will go on, for most. Today, I talked with patients like every other day, listened to their issues like every other day

However, today was a little different in that I realized I better be empathetic, because everyone has a struggle, a demon, a battle. Everyone.

Random Thoughts—14 December 2018

I'm not cut out to sit and do nothing. I allow myself the luxury of watching TV or general recreation only after all my work is done. This quirk has unfortunately interfered with fun on occasion, but it is also what helps me accomplish what I need to do.

Being stuck in a hospital as a patient is definitely not in my bailiwick . . . nobody got time for that.

Okay, so I was asked, what else can anyone like you take? This was in regard to ALS and cancer, and the answer is a central venous access port infection that has left septic emboli in both lungs and the potential for a heart infection called endocarditis. The plus side is my Christmas vacation just started a week earlier than planned and extended a few weeks later than planned. I'll possibly lose those pesky holiday pounds and will definitely be getting that ugly lumpy port out of my chest. I'll be beach ready, that's for sure. The downside is I can't lift anything heavier than 10lbs (like my coffee cup) for the remainder of the year. God's will be done. I love being around all the young nurses and doctors who are younger than my own kids.

Last day seeing patients. I would be taken to the hospital by ambulance.

I didn't know I was sick, but just a few hours later . . .

Random Thoughts While in Florida Living with Faith Based in Reality

To me, or should I say for me, faith allows us to see beyond physical limits. I have seen medical miracles that doctors from the various hospitals I have worked and even taught in cannot explain: cancers disappearing without medical intervention, and blind persons regaining their sight with no medical explanation.

I know centering oneself spiritually can have positive measurable effects on overall health, but I personally have found the Bible to be a useful How-To Manual or Instruction Guide. I have said it quite often that ALS does not define me; however, I do feel its effects. I could easily let the daily falls or the painful cramps that indicate more muscle death or the choking (the scariest symptom) really get to me. I could let the image in the mirror where once I saw eighteen-inch arms and legs so muscular a few pro athletes would compliment me and where I now see deteriorating flesh really get to me. I could let ALS steal the joy Darla Porter-Jines and I had on the beach by comparing it to the last time we were on the beach and I went a little farther than this time. I could let the images and negative voice (ALS steals relentlessly) gain a solid foothold on my psyche and become disillusioned so as to not try again later.

Everyone who is in my inner sanctum of friends knows I have dieted and exercised my entire adult life, but that is not enough. With ALS, there is nothing from the physical aspect that I have not done. This is the exact point where faith (notice I didn't say religion) can make a difference. Every page of the Bible stresses winning. We say sin, the Bible says salvation. We say sickness, the Bible says through Him we can find healing. We say death, and through the Bible, we can learn there is everlasting life. My favorite time of the year and the favorite holiday is upon us. I pray everyone who reads this finds a way to find Peace and Joy.

Random Thoughts and the Long Goodbye.

I'm sharing this because I have been given a gift of a diagnosis of ALS. It is a gift because anyone reading this could die tonight while still imagining you are immortal. I can guarantee you are not. In just a hundred years, everyone reading this will be dead. Guaranteed. I embrace my victim status by enjoying better parking, except at the Verizon Amphitheater. I enjoy my status by knowing every word of this is true. That is why I am having a blast dying as slowly as possible while knowing the truth.

Florida Pictures

Did two miles of sandy beach. Not the pace I used to do, but we had to stop and pick up seashells for the grand kiddos. Meika likes the ice cream beach treats here in Florida, and if she had opposable thumbs, she would feed herself . . . and another day full of memories in the book. ALS can stuff it.

ALS DX is a gift!

Random Thoughts

Since 9/11—Politics

Just because I have ALS doesn't preclude me from thinking about political issues. Ignoring politics will have people ruled by inferior intellects.

I've seen NEVER FORGET 9/11 . . . Really now. Oh, yeah, the Holocaust. NEVER FORGET . . . Yeah, right. What a joke.

It's been all but forgotten. There are elected officials that have said in public speeches that "some people did something" or that overt signs of National pride like the American flag or 9/11 Remembrance tributes are "offensive."

Since 9/11, I have watched patriotic Americans vilified. I have witnessed the American English language twisted through political correctness to the point that it's now considered hate speech to identify or say Muslim Islamic terrorists or identify the race of a suspect running from the scene of a crime or call an illegal alien just what they are: criminal invaders.

Through the political apathy of the general populace that is rampant in the majority of the voting public, we are now being ruled over (not represented) by a ruling class of intellectually inferior, historically ignorant, truth denying, factually challenged, reality and natural law denying collectivist statists. These progressive politicians are the result of a hundred-year push to destroy the constitution and reestablish a state religion of socialism, utilizing the divisive anti-American playbooks of Marx, Alinsky, Cloward, Piven, and the rest.

Our education system was subverted sixty years ago, as well as a huge percentage of the bureaucracy that is now called the Deep State (the unelected, unaccountable folks behind the curtain who wrote the rules they can ignore but we must adhere to).

Our experiment in self-governance is being destroyed from within. We have become a Balkanized, divided, hyphenated nation that no longer resembles a melting pot but instead a salad bowl.

On 12 September 2001, there was an inkling of unity that I prayed would last, but the MSM, which is an arm of the democrat party, has flagrantly through 90 percent negative coverage of any conservative representative including the President, along with the crime of omission of real truth and historical perspective, created an environment of division.

Be it race by the numbers, climate science, class envy, basic economics, the indoctrination of the general populace through their agenda-driven propaganda, it has allowed the acceptance (more like acquiescence) of the birth of criminal-supporting, terrorist-sympathizing, rule of law destroying, constitution shredding, hate-filled groups like CAIR (a co-conspirator of the 9/11 attack), BLM, ANTIFA here and ISIS abroad.

I pray we wake up to the double standards and outright hypocrisy demonstrated by the political ruling class on both sides of the aisle. I pray we see through the rhetoric designed to placate the apathetic and ignorant amongst us and again assert our God Given Freedoms. I pray those of us who still remember teach the next generation the truth of our Bill of Rights and where Rights truly come from (God, not government). I pray America Wakes Up. I pray America Never Forgets. Truly NEVER FORGETS. I pray America never appeases those who delivered us the Holocaust and the 9/11 Attacks.

If I have to explain that both are related, then you really need to read a few history books.

I for one will NEVER FORGET.

Plato is quoted and I'll paraphrase. You can ignore or be apathetic toward politics but remember, if you aren't interested in politics (politicians are always interested in controlling power over you). you do so at your own peril as your willing ignorance of what is going on will eventually cause you to be ruled over by inferior people.

I do not like either major party. I actually loathe both as they are just separate wings of the same bird. Our Founders realized this truth and also that the government may be limited. Large government becomes a living entity that takes and takes and will always be counted upon to waste as the individuals deciding where the money is spent are never responsible for the outcomes of their financial decisions. They just go to the trough and ask for more, with your time and life given over to your work, and then they determine what's a fair amount of your daily work to belong to them. Income tax to me is theft. If I take all of your labor, I have made you a slave. What percentage are you comfortable with?

We have been warned about the financial cliff, and every president in the last century has driven us closer. Bush II was derided by the Left and by me for fiscal irresponsibility. Obama doubled the national debt from all previous presidents and ushered in— in his own words—an era of lowered expectations (remember his shovel ready jobs programs weren't so shove-ready and that Trump doesn't have a magic wand speech). We are now, after tax cuts, giving the government record revenues (Kennedy was right, cutting taxes expands the economy and revenues), yet we are still spending near-record deficits yearly, adding to the national debt.

Politicians are presently promising programs (Green New Deal) that will spend more money than the entire world has. If we confiscate all the billionaires' and millionaires' combined fortunes, we could expect to run our government for a mere three months. Have you ever wondered where the shortfall would come from? You. Politicians sow class division and envy along with hundred years of empty promises of equal outcomes wrapped in socialist fairness and equal opportunity level playing field rhetoric.

There will always be poor. There will always be sloths. It is nature. It is human nature. Wake up.

Politicians will always promise security and safety. Hitler, Stalin, and Mao all promised safer children if their citizens would give up freedom and guns and became subjects. Our Founders knew this truth and made a Bill of Rights given to us by God instead of man so they couldn't be removed. They can be given away, though. All gun control is racist and always leads to genocide. Always. There are no gun control arguments that cannot be broken by the facts. Only fools believe guns are a problem or that politicians are concerned one iota about saving a single life. If you want sensible gun control, you are an ignorant fool. If you have an open mind, I know enough about this topic to prove my side of this convince you. Please believe me, I want safety and security too, and it is only maintained and achieved through freedoms.

Climate Change is a hoax! Same as class envy, gun control, and racial division the politicians have sold a whole generation on an indoctrinated lie. The science and facts along with common sense should convince any open-minded person of this. Only fools believe science is consensus. Only fools believe 97 percent of scientists believe Climate Change is real.

Why do so many spend $100 million for a job that pays $175k/year? It's not the salary. It's the power. Ever wonder where and why and how so many politicians you all know public servants get so rich? Pelosi, Romney, Kerry, Biden kids get no show jobs that pay millions for what? Access to the parents who sell foreign is aid.

Random Thoughts—Always be Thankful

Thankfulness is a well-visited topic of preachers and self-help gurus, *and* it is true, even when facing the a disease, financial problem, person relationship dilemma, etc. Case in point, me. I have ALS, and I there are no cures, and for me, there are no treatments available. I was told by one physician in the presence of my wife that the usual course is two to five years to death, but there are exceptions. I am thankful I am an exception. I just met a gentleman who had issues with balance last year, so he walked himself into the clinic and was diagnosed with ALS last September. Today, We talked for just a couple minutes, and I said I'll pray for him.

I couldn't help but think, "Man, oh, man, I'm lucky. I am a 100 percent disabled, yet, with effort, I can still saddle up and ride my motorcycle to Texas and back (already did it twice this year, and doing it again real soon).

I've adapted to its related realities but live as if there is a cure around the corner or my faith will cure it or others' prayers (I have a lot of well-wishers). about

I did feel guilty for quite a bit of time, not getting up daily and driving in demoralizingly life-sucking traffic to see my patients, my staff, and the other people I grew to love. They, on the other hand, continue to fight disease and save lives while telling me they miss me. I no longer feel guilt, but gratitude for the relationships built over the past four decades and the opportunity to enjoy the time allotted.

ALS, take a back seat.

Random Thoughts—Raising a Millennial Renaissance Man

I've been repeatedly asked by young men my son's age, "How did you do all that you do?"

An equal number have remarked that times are different, and that it must have been easier then, or worse yet, there's no way to do that today.

Nothing worthwhile is ever easy. It requires effort. Success is built upon like a building: brick by brick.

Renaissance men can be defined as a person with many talents or areas of knowledge. An outstandingly versatile, well-rounded person. The expression alludes to such Renaissance figures as Leonardo da Vinci, who performed brilliantly in many different fields.

I grew up with men who returned from WWII, each with great experiences to be taught and tremendous acumen in all areas of self-sufficiency and manliness. The world needs men like these, and those I strive to emulate.

There are many factors that contribute to creating Renaissance Men. Having two loving parents helps.

Ladies First: The benefits of a tiger mom and how modern moms can help their sons become the kind of man they can be proud of. Tiger moms don't hover and allow children to learn by falling down and getting back up. Tiger moms expect their children to get back up. Tiger moms don't want participation trophies. They want their child to succeed and win *real* trophies. My mother, a real tiger mom, told me quite adamantly that if I dishonored our family name or made bad decisions that ruined my future, that death would be a preferred outcome. She was serious and still is. Failure was never an option or quitting.

Here are some old school ideas my father passed on to me. My father grew up poor during the Great Depression, and it was the lessons of stifling poverty that taught him the value of hard work. Dad was the first in his family to graduate from high school and college, and this was the very definition of the American Dream: one's children going farther, accomplishing more, and climbing higher than the previous generation. Dad was a natural teacher who relished in providing jewels of wisdom while stimulating my brothers and me to continue to learn.

My earliest memories include my father stating, "When you go off to college . . ."

Note that he never said, "if."

Another memory was his admonition that we were all expected to move out once we completed high school and started college. He had an oft-repeated anecdote that he had certain expectations and milestones that he considered a must in order to obtain one's man card. Here's a short summary: Reading a map, defending one's principles verbally with logic and truth as well as physically with martial arts, acquiring the ability to pilot a small plane, ride a motorcycle, drive a car, speak a second language, and discuss the differences in writing styles between James Joyce and Ernest Hemingway, just to name a few.

The difference between Real Men and a Millennial Sheeple

What's manly about following the flock over a cliff? What's manly about not knowing what's going on not just in sports and entertainment but global politics? What's manly about referring to your significant other as bitches and hos instead of honoring your partners and being a man worth waiting for. What's manly about living off mommy and daddy well into your twenties, thirties, forties? What's manly about blaming others instead of taking responsibility for your actions and thoughts?

Random Thoughts—Millennial Must-See Movies

Hey, millennials. Do you know who John Wayne was? He was an actor and an American icon who made over two hundred movies. The reason I'm asking is he portrayed the quiet, courageous, tough, iconic cowboy, the type of man young American boys wanted to emulate. It really didn't matter the genre of film, he was himself in every one of those films. All young men deserve to become acquainted with him, and to that end, here are a few films to own or rent or download or just watch:

- Stagecoach
- She Wore a Yellow Ribbon

- The Quiet Man
- Rio Bravo
- The Searchers
- Hondo
- True Grit
- The Shootist
- The Man Who Shot Liberty Valance
- The Sands of Iwo Jima
- The Green Berets

There are more than a hundred others, but these represent why he was an icon and, again, what a man should act like.

While I'm thinking about this here are a few other films that serve as good examples of real men:

- To Hell and Back
- Bullitt
- Lawrence of Arabia
- Bridge over the River Kwai
- Dirty Harry
- Patton
- The Right Stuff
- Butch Cassidy and the Sundance Kid
- Tombstone

We Were Soldiers is a Mel Gibson movie.

Interestingly enough, every one of the films in the second group is based on true stories or real people. (Bullitt and Dirty Harry are actually based on a real San Francisco Inspector. Can you name him?).

I miss my real-life role models who were the WWII Greatest Generation. I'm tired of political correctness, victim mentality (there's nothing noble about being a victim), weak men, and situational ethics. Give me character-driven men who do the right thing and live by principles.

Random Thoughts—Veterans' Day

Happy Veterans; Day. Thank you all who have served and those serving now. Without the 1 percent of the population willing to serve, we would not be free to watch TV today and protest whatever is offending our sensibilities. Everything we do freely is a result of patriotic veterans willing to do the bidding of our elected government. Thank you, all.

Our family, the Jines Clan of Irish descent, has a long tradition of national service that was once celebrated at family gatherings like weddings. We would pray and thank our veterans and especially our family members who lost their lives in service to this nation. A ship's bell would be rung when the name was read. It was a tradition that would bring pride and one worthy of imitation.

Leaving a legacy for your family through our actions is a noble goal for one's lifetime. It is not stuff, money, and worldly goods (material things) that leave a positive mark when we die, but the changed minds and hearts of those we touched or guided that really are worth note. Living one's life as an example worthy of emulation should be a goal.

Serving more than yourself is worthy of respect and admiration.

I can think of only a handful of decisions one makes with one's life that can lead to a life well-lived. Who do you serve? What are you going to do with your life? Job? Career? Who will you spend it with? Pretty much every other decision you will ever make is secondary or has an effect on attaining your major goals. Smoking dope, taking drugs, excessive drinking, stealing, etc. are all choices that affect you reaching your potential. Signing the dotted line, taking the oath to serve our wonderful country, is a great step in living outside of yourself and leaving a legacy of a life well-lived.

Thank you again to all who have given me the freedom to choose what I have done, what I am doing now, and what may come.

Random Thoughts—Sunday after Thanksgiving and the Long Goodbye Continues

I am so thankful for this life and all that has made it what it is. I wouldn't know joy without feeling the deepest of hurts. I wouldn't appreciate the light without having been in darkness. The list goes on and on, seemingly without end. There will be an end. When I get to my end, I hope I don't have the baggage of regret. I don't want to carry a burden so heavy as to not have lived this life, this gift, completely. You know the old story of the biker that crashed into the heavenly gates completely worn out, having done everything he wanted to do until the end instead of being paralyzed by fear of failure.

Every one of us dies. Not everyone lives.

My friends in the special warfare community have a saying that the only easy day was yesterday. Tomorrow, I will be older. Tomorrow will offer opportunities that will be hard, and they will be even harder later down the road. My constant drum beat, Carpe Diem, is truth. Live now. Be thankful and forgive the past. We cannot change it, but we can change now. You will never be in a better position to make a positive change in your life than now. Not yesterday. Sorry, no redos. Tomorrow isn't here yet.

I'm so lucky to have my girl in my life. I could not ask for a better partner, wingman, cheerleader, and one to give perspective. I hit a homer while batting way out of my league. It's because I tried.

Random Thoughts—Christmas Movies

I love Christmas movies!

There was a time when all Christmas movies were about the religious meaning—the reason for the season. Classics like *A Christmas Carol,* Dickens' classic that shaped the way we have celebrated Christmas for over 175 years, have been remade several times. Each following the book reminds us that our spirit must go out amongst our fellow men. We can find forgiveness, we can change for good (Wicked reference), we can make a difference. Of all the versions, my favorite is the 1951 Alistair Sim version. Watch this with an open heart and see how Scrooge's childhood trauma and lost love shaped him. Then watch as he learns to forgive then is forgiven and how we can all keep Christmas every day. 1984's George C. Scott's version is a close runner up. The rest is passable.

James Stewart revived his career after WWII with his role in *It's a Wonderful Life*. This is a classic about the significance of one life. His contemplated suicide, like any suicide, would have a ripple effect that the suicide victim may never have intended.

Hallmark . . . what can I say? Today's Christmas classic is all about personal romance and, in most cases, has lost its biblical and therefore spiritual connection. Yes, I always seem to cry that ugly cry when I watch one alone, and they are addictive, but I don't have the same deep personal connection as these characters are not me. They are not speaking to my inner self looking for the meaning of life and not just a little romance.

Hallmark Synopsis
Girl comes from the big city to escape the stress of big corporate life. Her boyfriend has not made the commitment, or she's single. She runs into a guy that she doesn't like at first. He is recently widowed and has a cute kid. There's a black guy sitting in the diner or a black guy who is her demanding but understanding big corporate boss. There's a conflict that eventually requires a girl and a single guy to work together. They fall in love, and it starts to snow in the end.

Christmas Vacation. What a departure from tradition. Very funny, and I really believe there are many misguided Clark Griswalds that love their family. I watch this every year and have the lingerie sales clerk's autographed picture. Thanks, Nicolette Scorsese (not related to Martin).

The more secular and the more devolved we become, the farther we move from the reason for the holiday. This is where Lethal

Weapon and Die Hard come to mind. That's what I was thinking while drinking my morning Joe. That and Impeachment.

PS: I love watching the hero of Nakatomi Plaza.

Random Thoughts—ALS sucks and I Allowed It into My Head
17 December 2019

We all like to put our best life forward on social media. Occasionally, we have friends who put their drama out there, as if any of us really want to see it or even care. Most of the time when we read a post where it's a nonstop bitchfest or never-ending pity party, we can at least feel, "Thank God it is not me!"

Where's the lesson? What positive contribution can be taken from a rant?

We all have struggles and bills and jobs and stress, whether you are a billionaire running the greatest country on Earth or the stock clerk forced to clean a homeless person's feces from the aisle of a San Francisco grocery store. We all got battles. This has been illustrated here in my previous Random Thoughts, essays, and thousands of self-help books.

Today was one of those days. You know, the kind that lets you know early on that you'd be better off going back to bed, or if you are Rodney Dangerfield, maybe just start drinking now.

ALS decided to make its presence known by interfering with my ability to remove snow from a windshield, and even before that, just saying no to walking to my car without falling first. I'm used to falling, now. Far more painful than the deep bruising and jammed or sprained or strained joints is the realization that this is my norm. I needed to get ready to go see my doctor, but instead, there I was lying in a puddle of slush unable to get up. So much for being all cleaned up and on my way. Instead, I had to get all cleaned up again. I'm used to doing that too. Anyone who knows me knows being punctual is important, and I don't like to rush nor being rushed. Everything I now attempt to do takes more time.

Estimating how long the most mundane of tasks will take is no longer a recognizable routine. Button a shirt, ten to twenty minutes. Button the 501 fly . . . dear God. Putting on a pair of socks, two to three minutes. Get the picture? I'm still guilty of thinking I'm normal, then reality slaps me like Cher slapping Nick Cage in *Moonstruck*. Pow.

After this morning, Darla was there, as always, saying the right things, being a source of encouragement and strength, not letting me or my perfectionist nature get the best of me. I was miserable, I'm sure, blaming God, blaming fate, angry I was unable to get out on time, angry I wasn't getting my way, angry I'm not who I have been, angry, angry, angry. All this time, Darla says all she sees is this strong guy, her heart filled with the joy of the season and a filter that allows her to see beyond my limitations and to that guy she fell in love with.

I really wish I was him all the time. Today, I was feeling neither strong nor positive. I allowed myself to feel sorry for myself. It is not an admirable behavior.

Random Thoughts—Winter Solstice Office Appreciation
Enjoying coffee on a Solstice morning. Already posted some political stuff and feeling grateful for all the blessings that keep coming my way. We live in the freest nation on the planet. People are lining up to get in, not leave. Compared to thirty to forty years ago, we have more clean air, less poverty, less violent crime (despite media lies), more good and less bad. I'm blessed to wake up and look out to a view that most would find beautiful and breathtaking. I am weathering this whole retirement storm not wanting for anything. I have my health. Thanks to a lifetime of organic and intense workouts, I'm still walking way past my doctor's expiration date.

Thankful for my wife's devotion and her hard work, taking up the slack I am passing along. I'm thankful for the blessings that hard work and right decisions afforded me at home and at work.

My Southampton coffee mug is a reminder that I owe so much to a staff that made and continues to make my vision of healthcare successful. Healthcare is a business, and it is a privilege to be trusted by so many. Having a supportive staff makes providing necessary and high-quality care possible. From the top to bottom and bottom to top, the entire staff works together with shared goals of doing everything humanly possible to do it right. Katherine Weyhaupt has been the rock in all the administrations necessary to allow the providers the opportunity to practice low volume high-quality care. Her tireless work ethic has been recognized by local charities, the public health dept, and even the federal funding sources that are in charge of quality assurance and financial considerations. Doctors can't be good doctors if they are consumed with every penny coming in and out. Doctors need a trusted administrator and Katherine is our manager and friend.

I'm blessed to have fellow providers doctors and hygienists that are top tier providers. By the level of continuing education by their own self-starting initiative and their personal drive to excellence, they have continued a tradition of being providers not only to the public but to many on the top docs in St. Louis. My friend Joe C. Paulfrey always said, "It ain't bragging when it's just a fact!"

I'm so blessed to have the best (other guys have openly tried to hire away many of my staff) assistants like Tracy Brust, Tina, Julie, and Kelly, making what the providers do possible. This team and life in general are a blessing, and I'm thankful today.

Random Thoughts—Christmas Eve Past, Present, and Future
I'm sitting here watching *A Christmas Carol*, the 1951 version starring Alistair Sim, with Darla. This is my favorite version, though I do like them all, whether it is 1938's Reginald Owen or Capt. Piccard's version or even General Patton . . . just kidding, Patrick Stewart and George C Scott respectively. I've watched this particular film and the play at the Fox. This includes several times during

the season. I started watching this with my grandfather Charlie and my dad, and it has been a tradition I've carried on, even forcing my kids to watch.

This story tugs my heart is so many ways, I can barely see the screen while watching it. Wouldn't it be nice if we all could be invited to replay our pasts and garner an understanding of past pains from another mature point of view. How wonderful could this world be if we understood the magic from this story is real. We must let go of those past hurts, no matter how bad and whose fault. Holding onto the pain and reliving the past only ensures we never grow or flourish. If we embrace the spirit of this season and keep it 365 days instead of just one, imagine how bright our future could be.

Christmas Day is a few minutes away, and I wish all a very Merry Christmas.

As children, it was all about unwrapping the magic we found under the tree. As a parent and grandparent, I know the magic is in the giving.

I would give anything to have less stuff and more happy memories with my son and daughter. I accumulated a lot of stuff, and while it's great having the accouterments of a certain amount of success, I'm looking at life differently now, especially given the gift of a diagnosis that means there is a certainty to an expiration date or the impending consequences of said diagnosis, I have mental clarity and the ability to prioritize better than before.

I know we all die. I know there are no guarantees. You and I can easily get hit by that proverbial bus tomorrow. We all live with a certain ability to rationalize life to ourselves. We all live with a certain amount of teen spirit (sorry, Nirvana) that holds we have invincibility and immortality as long as we think and act a certain way and never ever give up. It's just when you are dealt a handful of lousy cards or lemons that you either hold, fold, bluff, or make lemonade, meaning we all deal with life's curveballs individually.

There is no real right or wrong way. Some quit, some fight to the end, some do a combination of both, and others even choose to Carpe you know what out of their Diem . . . Hey, get back on track, here. This is a Christmas post.

I'm more patient, now. I drive slower and am more thankful. I'm glad God has given me this time to ask for forgiveness. I'm glad that Darla and I are doing as many activities as possible with plans to ride cross country at least three times in the coming year. This Christmas, I pray you all find a reason to renew your faith. When you see me limping along, remember that miracles happen and God is not through with me yet. When you see me limping along, have faith in the one who made the blind see, the lame walk, and who overcame death for all of us. Please be grateful, please forgive, and please be kinder and try in 2020 to live Christmas all year.

Random Thoughts—30 December 2019
What can I say except I am one of those guys who is so lucky that when I'm asked, "How are you doing?" I reply, "Better than I deserve," and I am not lying.

This year marked a new life, as I saw and treated my last patient in December 2018. I was doing great dealing with the ALS diagnosis I've had for half a decade. I had already outlived the average lifespan of Lou Gehrig's patients worldwide and scored off the chart on the ALS function scale. My dexterity and strength measurements were at the highest end of the normal scale with a top one certain grip strength, etc. I had been doing my own regimen of regular exercise (forty-five years, three to five days a week) and a very healthy diet. Then, I got the surprise of an aggressive cancer diagnosis, despite a normal exam and no symptoms.

So, 2019 started with surgery, radiation, and chemotherapy, and all the while, a plan of returning to my clinical practice and being a clinical mentor. Well, it took all year to actually beat the side effects of cancer treatment. While I was dealing with cancer,

I had to stop many of the routine treatments for the ALS. The ALS has taken the opportunity to manifest itself by taking my balance, dexterity, and strength very rapidly, necessitating assistance in walking: wheelchair and scooters when not using a walker or two canes.

2019 was still a great year. Darla (she is my hero) and I traveled to Bandera, Tx. for our motorcycle club's (Reguladores LEMC) winter national meeting, then straight over to Florida for beach time and recuperation. We rode down to Ragin Cajun in Lafayette, La., another Regulardores LEMC event, then we were off to Gulf Shores. I rode with friends, brothers, and sisters to the last Rolling Thunder in Washington DC (thankfully, it won't be the last) and then back to Baltimore to visit a new Chapter of our MC with founder and friend Richard Max Maxwell. Darla and I rode up to the Canadian border to visit the Gichigami Chapter of Reguladores and then down to Corpus Christi, Tx. for our club's Bikers for Boobs Breast Cancer fundraiser. We rode up to Bristol, Wi. to visit my son and family, and I did a couple of weekend fundraisers up north again with brothers and sisters during the 9/11 remembrance time.

We are blessed to be able to recuperate while getting out, and my hopes are that I will eventually get back to work.

We took a cruise to the Bahamas, and even though I've treated sleep apnea, I was introduced to new technology so revolutionary as to put the old sleep appliances including CPAP into the backseat and eventually completely away. I was so impressed with the science and then the life-saving necessity for this new therapy that I brought it back to Southampton Dental, where it was determined my staff will get certified over the next year in the newest Sleep Medicine. This will save lives and immeasurably improve the quality of life of all our patients suffering from a plethora of medical and dental conditions. This therapy will improve not only sleep but has been shown in literature to decrease mortality, hypertension, diabetes, PANDAS, and so much more. I'm proud of the commitment everyone is making and especially Drs. Cal Harmon and Michael Czeschin for the sacrifices in time and energy as they become certified in sleep medicine.

Oh, well, this Random Thoughts has to end as my waiting room time is up, and the doctor will be seeing me now.

Peace and Happy New Year.

PS: Carpe Diem because Memento Mori. Live a life that outlives you!

PPS. Thank you, Dr. Mathew Worth. Dr. Worth is a Chiropractic Physician and post-doctorally trained neurologist who lectures all around the world on the rehabilitation of neurological conditions. I was referred to him by one of my internists with the recommendation that this guy gets results. I have personally seen him get people out of wheelchairs and kids who received brain injuries that both big Children's Hospital said were hopeless and forever uneducable. Instead, they are back in regular school and thriving. I am so thankful he and his staff at Missouri Brain and Spine Rehabilitation Center have been my care provider. I am so blessed.

Happy New Year 2020 This is NOT the end.

ALS Diagnosis Was a Gift

When I started to write this story, I said it's a choice. How we react and choose to fight any diagnosis like ALS starts with a decision. I have lived looking at reality and believing in reality, not something I hoped for or something theoretical like utopian pipe dreams. I'm sharing this because I have been given a gift of a diagnosis of ALS. It is a gift because anyone reading this could die tonight while still imagining you are immortal. I can guarantee you are not. In just a hundred years, everyone reading this will be dead. Guaranteed. I embrace my victim status by enjoying better parking, except at the Verizon Amphitheater. That is why I am having a blast dying as slowly as possible while knowing the truth.

COVID-19 2020 Edit and additional RANDOM THOUGHTS

Since submitting this daily journal of Random Thoughts and Activities the 2020 COVID-19 World Pandemic Panicked the world into standstill. Lockdowns, forced quarantines as well as self quarantine measures gripped the headlines and in all that science was politicized and freedoms were lost. As this was sorting itself out economies were crashed leading to potentially more death and destruction than the disease itself. Life still goes on and will do while the shutdowns were in full effect I had the opportunity to add to this book by inserting my clinical education writings just to fill in a few more pages.

One thing to note about the next few paragraphs about COVID-19 is how the narrative changed as I garnered further information and as the political football game surrounding this virus was becoming more clear as the science offered more questions than answers.

CORONAVIRUS

I HAVE BEEN DELUGED WITH QUESTIONS. HERE IS WHAT I KNOW.

80% of people who are infected with COVID-19 will have minimal to moderate symptoms. Most cases in healthy people will resolve in 3 days.
Nature Medicine, March 16, 2020).
SINCE ITS MILD MANY CARRY IT FOR 10-40 DAYS. SO YOU CAN BE CONTAGIOUS WAY LONGER THAN YOU ARE SICK. THATS WHY THE GOVERNMENT WANTS YOU TO STAY HOME WHEN YOU ARE SICK. (The Lancet, March 11, 2020)

The World Health Organization (WHO) gave the new coronavirus the name "COVID-19" on February 11, 2020, and declared it a pandemic on March 10, 2020. That's less than a month! A review of 22 studies on similar human coronaviruses such as SARS (Severe Acute Respiratory Syndrome coronavirus), MERS (Middle East Respiratory Syndrome coronavirus) and HCoV (endemic human coronaviruses) finds that COVID-19 is not more severe than many flu viruses (J of Hosp Infect, Feb 6, 2020).

COVID-19 is incredibly contagious because no human has been shown to have been infected with this virus before this year ever. There can be no immunity because no one has ever had this. ITS NOT BEEN SHOWN IN ANY SCIENTIFIC STUDY TO HAVE BEEN A BIOENGINEERED MILITARY WEAPON.

The current working theory is this started in some animal and then was transmitted to humans and was first identified in Wuhan, China. The doctor who discovered this died. He was young and healthy but allergic to lead poisoning. (The Chinese charged him with spreading rumors. The Chinese drug their feet on reporting this so stop blaming the USA and the current administration) It is now being transmitted from person to person in countries all over the world.

COVID-19 can infect anyone because as I stated at top no one had ever had this. No one was immune until this first appeared in early 2020. Most people do not have any symptoms or have only mild symptoms the majority won't know the difference from a common cold. The most likely to become ill are folks over 65 years old and those with other diseases or a weakened immune system are more likely to have serious symptoms, severe disease and even death. Older people are at higher risk for complications because as we age our immune systems decrease in efficiency. This is another reason resistance training helps because the more muscle we have the better our immune systems work. (People with healthier lifestyles fair better).

Among the people in the U.S. who have died from COVID-19, almost all have been in their 70s, 80s or 90s. So far, the youngest known fatality was a man in his 40s (New York Times, Mar 14, 2020).

HOW DOES THIS SPREAD

COVID-19 is spread by contagious respiratory droplets, primarily from person-to-person. sneezing or cough, causes the virus to be suspended in the air for up to three hours. COVER YOUR MOUTH WITH YOUR SLEEVES PLEASE! TISSUES ARE BETTER BECAUSE YOU CAN DISCARD THE TISSUE!!!!If you sneeze into your hand AVOID TOUCHING YOUR FACE. Sneezing on your hands and then touch a door handle.....it can be SPREAD TO and FROM from surfaces such as door handles, furniture, clothes or any other object that you may touch.

Because many will never know they are sick many will spread this without knowing. COVID-19 has an incubation period of about 2-10 days after exposure to an infected person or surface. During this time you call spread it to or get it from others. The virus initially lives in the nose and throat and then goes down into the lungs. Early symptoms include shortness of breath, fever, and feeling sick.

COVID-19 Infected people keep the live virus for an average 20 days and can continue to be contagious for eight to 37 days, even if they have no symptoms (The Lancet, March 11, 2020).

There are no known effective treatments. Most people with normal immune systems are likely to get rid of the virus and feel better within a few days. Current flu meds may help symptoms.

WHO IS AT INCREASED RISK

ANYONE WITH IMMUNE SYSTEM ISSUE! : a history of heart attacks, cancers, diabetes, lung disease, auto-immune disease, chronic infection or any other serious illness. So far, of the most seriously ill COVID-19 patients, 30 percent had high blood pressure, 19 percent had diabetes, and 8 percent had serious heart disease. People with an existing lung disease (asthma, bronchitis, emphysema, and so forth) are at high risk for complications.

COVID-19 CAUSES DEATH FROM RESPIRATORY FAILURE. The majority of deaths occur after the virus spreads from the sinuses and throat to the lungs of already ill patients.

WHAT SHOULD YOU DO

WASH YOUR HANDS. USE ALCOHOL BASED SANITIZER

USE SANITIZER ON ANY HARD surfaces such as metal, glass or plastic can remain contagious for about 10 days at normal room temperatures, and at near-freezing temperatures they can remain contagious for about 18 days. If a suspect package is shipped to you, you may want to wait for several days before opening it. Most virus particles break down in minutes or hours outside a living host, and you are far more likely to acquire the virus directly from another person.

FACE MASKS ARE USELESS FOR PREVENTION ON HEALTHY PEOPLE

FACE MASKS should be used on infected patients to protect others! FACE MASKS are almost useless for preventing infection! Health care workers and other people who are frequently exposed to sick people should wear masks.

STAY HOME

All people with weak immune systems should avoid crowds, hospitals, and any unnecessary exposure to potentially sick people.

If you are at high risk of any complications of COVID-19 as described you may want to follow even stricter avoidance or self-isolation measures to reduce your chances of exposure.

CLOSING UP SHOP

Federal, state and local governments, health departments, schools and businesses are issuing orders and recommendations for cancellations, closures, social distancing, travel restrictions and other measures to help stop the spread of COVID-19.

This is a serious pandemic but this is not a doomsday apocalypse. Sit back relax and breath. Then wash your hands at least 20 seconds. Disinfect everything you touch with alcohol. Don't sneeze and cough without covering up. Protect others. Using tissue is best a sleeve second best. Stay in if you are old or old and sick. Stay home if you are sick. This will pass but for Gods sake please stop panicking and overwhelming our hospitals with needless visits.

Dr. Denzel D. Jines

PS please take a look at what's going on behind the scenes. This is a political football being used to wreck the economy more than a zombie apocalypse. This virus is again no more deadly than the others I listed above. It's just scary because it's the first time to infect people and therefore there isn't widespread immunity.

COVID-19 TREATMENT AS OF EARLY 19 MARCH 2020

So far here is what I have found in REAL JOURNALS. Yesterday I mentioned the anti-malarial that's called chloroquine. It's relatively safe and can be given to pregnant women. Since yesterday this is what I know:

As of right now there are no drugs that have been proven to treat COVID-19.

Chloroquine phosphate, was safe and effective in shortening the course and decreasing symptoms in patients suffering from COVID-19 pneumonia (Biosci Trends, Mar 16, 2020;14(1):72-73). I mentioned this one yesterday. It's been around for a long time and fairly safe. It comes from a Chinese study.

The World Health Organization (WHO) has started trials for this drug and three others.

1. the antimalarial drug chloroquine
2. the antiviral drug remdesivir (Gilead)
3. a combination of two HIV drugs, lopinavir and ritonavir (AbbVie)
4. lopinavir and ritonavir plus interferon beta

So far, one study from China reports that lopinavir and ritonavir are not effective in treating COVID-19 infections (NEJM, Mar 18, 2020).

KEEP THOSE PRAYERS GOING AND HOPES HIGH THAT A CURE IS FOUND OR AT LEAST ONE EFFECTIVE TREATMENT.

COVID19 101 SHELTER IN PLACE WHY????

If this isn't the deadliest virus why is there so much panic? Why do we have to stay in if we are young and probably won't get sick?

WE ARE TRYING TO AVOID BECOMING ITALY!

This virus is unlike others in the fact that there was no immunity in population because it was new. Therefore EVERYONE can get it.

So what happened in Italy?
Almost everyone got it at once.

EXAMPLE:
There are 10 hospitals and there are 1000 people and each hospital can see 10 patients at a time.

So now an infection COVID19 comes along. All 1000 people are going to get it.

10 people get it in a week....no problem there's room.

All 1000 get it all at once and...no room at the inn. Over worked staffs get sick too, not enough docs and nurses to treat, not enough ventilators etc. ITALY ALL OVER AGAIN HERE.

SOLUTION: WASH HANDS , AVOID CROWDS, QUIT BEING SELF CENTERED NARCISSISTIC TOILET PAPER HOARDING, OVERLY SENSITIVE,EASILY OFFENDED JERKS. TAKE CARE OF EACH OTHER AND BE KIND. BE PATIENT.

COVID-19 Update. 30 March 2020

I'm in process of final editing two books that will be out later this year. I have not been watching the Facebook feed of late except for skimming a few friendly faces. Today I read one comment and it took my attention away for about a minute to rant. Now I'm back and here's a few cogent thoughts on COVID19

Like usual the USA is now again a world leader(if you trust China and India reporting)but this isn't good. We are number 1 now in this pandemic. COVID19 was first reported by the Chinese in Dec 2019 AFTER IT WAS OUT OF CONTROL! What's interesting is countries bordering or near China started screening patients and quarantining them early. Taiwan, S. Korea and Vietnam did what was smart and isolated individuals suspected of being ill to slow the epidemic down. It's the only ways.

When Trump was first advised he ordered the travel restrictions that have potentially saved us. He ordered the restrictions within one week! The DEMOCRAT media and politicians cried RACISM.

Democrats like I was going to name a few but ALL said he was racist. Mayor of NYC said in February and again in March to go party and go parade. The Health dept of NYC said nothing to fear, it's all under control! Watch the quotes.

So party on as advised by the Speaker of the House even in early March the democrat politicians said head out to Mardi Gras and spring break and St. Patrick's Day and whoops.......NOW ITS ALL TRUMPS FAULT.

I don't like either political party. I have pointed out the weaknesses of both while pushing politically for increased freedom. As a healthcare provider who practices using evidence based therapies founded in science I look for the truth not political pandering for funding nor do I look for special rights due to my minority status. JUST THE FACTS.

STOP WITH THE ORANGE MAN, RACIST, XENOPHOBIC, CLASS AND RACE DIVISION BULLSHIT. START INTELLIGENT CONVERSATIONS USING REAL DEMONSTRABLE FACT. NO HE ISN'T ELOQUENT. HE SCREWED AROUND...ALOT. SO DID EVERY OTHER LEADER BIG DEAL.

RACHEL MADDOW HAS BEEN SHOWN ALONG WITH EVERY CNN AND MSNBC ANCHOR TO OUTRIGHT LIE. THE LIST IS EXHAUSTING SEEING THEM PROVEN WRONG. IF YOU ARE TOO INTELLECTUALLY CHALLENGED TO FIND THE TRUTH QUIT OFFERING THEIR LIES AS YOUR OWN THOUGHTS! I am sick of liberal hyperbole wrapped up in vitriolic hubris.

Obama cut CDC funding NOT orange man.

Pelosi said Orange man fiddled while not addressing COVID 19. She referenced Emperor Nero fiddling while Rome burned. Yet she is clearly on camera encouraging people to ignore Trump.

Now go have a good day. I'm going to keep the update short so you can all go take on the challenges of the day. Bye bye.

Quarantine Journal Day......the same as yesterday. Science and politics clash with freedom at stake so I think I'll watch some tv since actually doing some of the work needed around here is impossible since I cannot under orders leave the house. She thinks I'll get corona.

Sooooo what to do. I saw many reviews of a few NetFlix shows. AMAZING. OZARK. We are watching the first season and it's well written and one of those shows where we feel sorry for the good guys because there are very few. The kids. The Preacher. The Bar and restaurant and real estate agent.....everyone else is badddddd. The series premiere throws some major curves thanks to the shows narrator Marty's business partner Bruce. Then all of this is happening as Marty's personal life is going down the toilet faster than a corona virus tainted Deviled egg that's been room temp too long. It's compelling. Like Homeland and Ray Donovan this is gritty.

COVID-19 UPDATE.

I posted a COVID-19 (101) last week and here's some updated treatment protocols after a quick review of ongoing research and a couple RANDOM THOUGHTS.

COVID-19 has been shown so far to have been similar in severity to other flu viruses. When looking at the thousands of deaths caused yearly by the others case in point 2009 Swine flu in the USA. Here's what's different, no one is immune and therefore this is extremely contagious. There was until now no cases and it was the WHO that named COVID-19 on 10 February 2020. WHO called it a pandemic 10 March 2020.

THE PRESIDENT OF THE USA DID THE ONE THING ALL ALL EVERY EXPERT SAYS IS ESSENTIAL TO SLOWING A PANDEMIC. He restricted travel within a week of learning there was a new flu back in January 2020. So while he took great heat and was called a racist, xenophobic idiot by the democrats and their minions the press who have got it wrong he was right. Nancy Pelosi the Mayor of NYC and the Health Director of the state of NYC are on video encouraging people to get out an mingle as late as middle March 2020!

My post earlier still stands as to who is most at risk and recommendations about preventing spread. Go to CDC or WHO for updates there.

Here are latest treatment facts:

These are case reports and no double blind placebo controlled large patient based research studies but reports from the trenches.

Hydroxychloroquine (Plaquenil) was found to be significantly more potent than chloroquine in killing COVID-19 (Clinical Infectious Diseases, March 9, 2020). Treating physicians using a loading dose of 400 mg twice daily of hydroxychloroquine given orally, followed by a maintenance dose of 200 mg given twice daily for four days found it reached three times the potency of chloroquine given 500 mg twice daily for five days.

Dr Stephen Smith, of East Orange, NJ, reports that he has treated 72 COVID-19 patients, most of whom were morbidly obese (over 300 pounds), diabetic or prediabetic, with hydroxychloroquine (Plaquenil is a newer anti malarial drug than chloroquine) and azithromycin(antibiotic that kill bacteria) for five days. None of the patients required intubation (a ventilator). This followed a Seattle study of 40 patients, of whom half were diabetic or prediabetic, using the same drug combination. None had to be put on a ventilator, but two of the 40 patients developed irregular heartbeats.

A French study found that five days of this same drug combination completely eliminated the virus from the nose and throat in 30 patients, compared to 10 percent in the control group and 50 percent of those receiving only chloroquine (J of Antimicrobial Agents, March 17, 2020).

Chloroquine(anti malarial drug) has been reported to reduce symptoms and hasten recovery in several small studies (Biosci Trends, Mar 16, 2020;14(1):72-73). You can see from the NJ report that Plaquenil May be more potent.

A Chinese unpublished study of 62 patients showed a marked reduction in fever and cough in patients taking hydroxychloroquine.

Dr. Vladimir Zelenko of Monroe, NY, reports that he has successfully treated patients with a five-day course of hydroxychloroquine 200 mg twice a day, azithromycin 500 mg once a day, and zinc sulfate 220mg once a day, he has not yet published this but he is reporting this to the media.

ITS TIME TO STOP THE POLITICS, REPORT THE FACTS AND MAINTAIN FREEDOM. WE NEED TO GET BACK TO TO WORK. THE GOVERNMENT HAS ALREADY BROKEN THE PIGGY BANK. THE STIMULUS WAS FULL OF PORK SPENDING AND KICKBACKS THAT HAD NOTHING TO DO WITH HELPING THIS CRISIS.

WE CAN NOT SPEND OURSELVES INTO PROSPERITY. PAYING PEOPLE MORE THAN THEY EARN WHILE WORKING IS A PRESCRIPTION TO RUIN. THE DEBT TRAIN AND THE FINANCIAL CLIFF ARE CLOSER THAN EVER.

D. D. Jines DMD,MD.

Quarantine Diary early April 2020

Meika perched upon her throne in the sunroom surveying her domain.

Quarantine day 20. FYI 99.6% of the people who get COVID19 recover.

Every model that predicted the deaths are being revised down. Some by a factor of 8 times!!!!

One model now showing 50% of USA may have also been exposed.

Relax, breath, then pray and be kind.

COVID UPDATE. 4/6/20

I was asked how do I know if I got it? What's it look like?

Many who are infected, may have no symptoms at all. Symptoms usually develop 2 to 10 days after you acquire the virus(most within 5-7 day range). Symptoms may come on fast and initially present like the flu but go on to develop fever, cough, and shortness of breath. The virus lives in your nose and throat (points of entry) leading to sniffles and sore throat and then can go down into your lungs. You may also suffer belly cramps and diarrhea, and the virus can be transmitted in the stool (Gastroenterology, accepted Feb 27, 2020, not yet published).

COVID-19 is dangerous because it can infect your lungs and fill them up with mucus to smother you(Think of a sponge filled with water. That's the lungs of a COVID patient). COVID can cause your immunity to become over active so that the same cells and chemicals that normally attack germs starts to damage normal healthy (called "cytokine storm"). This hasn't changed since the beginning....the "majority" of people most likely to suffer severe consequences from this infection include people over 65 and those who have diabetes, high blood pressure, heart disease, lung disease, kidney disease, asthma, immune defects, HIV, bleeding or clotting defects, or auto-immune diseases. Possible effects on pregnancy or unborn children are not yet known. Some patients appear to suffer long term heart damage after COVID-19 infections (Lancet, March 28, 2020;395:11054-1062).

Earlier I posted that infected people keep the live virus for an average of 20 days (Am J of Resp and Crit Care Med, Mar 23, 2020), and can continue to be contagious for up to 37 days, even if they have no symptoms (The Lancet, March 11, 2020). Sputum samples remain positive up to 39 days and stool samples for 13 days (Annals of Internal Medicine, March 30, 2020).

So far as treatments.....NONE APPROVED; HOWEVER, there are plenty of unpublished(some in pre print) that are showing good results with the same drugs mentioned in the last update.

Political Warning

Saul Alinsky said,"Never let a crisis go to waste. Always accuse your opponent(Patriotic, Conservative Americans) of what you are doing."

I saw some of my favorite liberals calling Trump dumb because he asked the difference between HIV and HPV. Left at that with no context then it may come across to any non critical thinker that the a President isn't sure which one causes AIDS and which one is causing Cervical and throat cancers. Trump was asking about vaccines and why HIV has been more difficult create a vaccine for compared to HPV.

Every model used for climate change AND COVID have been proven wildly wrong. As I mentioned this morning the new models are showing decreases up to 8 times different than original models.

We have doctors who are politicians more so than doctors. They are the "experts"and guiding the response.

They have secure positions and don't have an interest in how this or any crisis effects the average citizen or business owner.

I am only passing on the peer reviewed materials not opinion except my questioning of the faulty models. The models are only as good as the data input and unfortunately we don't have all the answers and therefore I'm reluctant to blindly follow suggestions that cripple economies or freedom.

WAKE UP.
Dr. D. D. JINES.

COVID and POLITICS and the CYA.

Yesterday Dr. Fauci said on TV that Trump was slow to react because he didn't take advise soon enough. He said people died because Trump didn't close off borders etc..Timeline proves Fauci stated COVID19 was NOTHING TO WORRY ABOUT 21-26 Jan. MARCH 9 FAUCI stated GO ON A CRUISE! Trump had already closed travel to China while the experts were saying we are safe there's nothing to worry about. The revision of the model numbers prove their modes are wrong. 95% wrong. Wrong wrong wrong. Trump was slammed for following the experts advise by the experts!

Dr. D. D. Jines.

This is not a personal attack. His response to Al Sharpton on TV Easter was politically biased. I am showing that during this fluid situation Trump counted on Fauci as the expert who advised Trump 19 Feb this is a low risk virus. He said he Chinese are transparent.

He said that closing NYC or Chicago would be draconian and impossible. I personally like him he has been a leader against infectious disease for decades but he's also a political animal and that bias requires questions.

The democrats in collusion with China and WHO and a biased CDC have used faulty models to scare the USA into a Depression. The facts and reality don't match the narrative. Yes COVID is scary but more people have died of the flu this season. The spike in the curve or the gradual infection curve still means the same number of cases. Falsely inflating COVID death numbers doesn't help me believe the CDC has the best tract record nor do I have faith in models any longer. If you are in a risk group isolate and if you are sick stay home but the majority of the population should now go outside.

RANDOM THOUGHTS...WHO IS AT MOST RISK FOR COVID-19 DEATH.

For those that read my RANDOM THOUGHTS you'll recognize to the point of nausea that I stress living a healthy lifestyle. I've spent an adult lifetime practicing healthcare at the intersection of Dentistry and Medicine. I've advised countless patients, students and friends about everything from good internal and external hygiene to how dentistry and in particular dental disease exacerbates medical conditions. If you've read my RANDOM THOUGHTS you've witnessed my passion explaining we don't have a healthcare crisis as much as a health crisis in America. I've cited a plethora of peer reviewed studies that state much of the medicine prescribed today is to counteract the side effects of medicines that are prescribed and taken for illnesses caused by unhealthy lifestyles.

The current COVID crisis and the freedom destroying unConstitutional lockdown are a symptom not just of politicizing a virus but also a demonstration of why I have for my entire career stressed lifestyle changes as a means to remain healthy and free instead of blithely following the modern model of treatment of symptoms. THERE ARE NO MAGIC PILLS TO CURE YOUR ILLS.

What was this you just read? How did politics and COVID and Freedom and lifestyle all come together. Simple if you want to remain free and live life to its fullest your health is one of if not your most important assets.

40% of the general population in the USA is now obese! That's right nearly half of this nation has a BMI over 30. Wait wait wait what does being obese or merely overweight have to do with COVID? Before we get there let me explain about getting fat. It helps to understand this so that we can all then make the necessary changes to keep us less susceptible to illness, infections etc.

Any calorie you eat that you do not burn off turns into fat. It doesn't matter where the calorie comes from. One extra calorie from fat, protein, carbohydrates will turn into fat if it's not utilized to provide energy. Our bodies are efficient at converting extra calories into extra pounds and inches. Two thirds of all of us are genetically predisposed to become diabetics because diabetics actually did better during the times of famine our ancestors went through. I guess you can blame genes, but only so far.

So now here's a little more technical science on getting fat.

When your body fails to respond to the hormone leptin, which is a hormone that tells you to STOP eating you eat excess calories because leptin tells you that you are full. Extra calories are turned into fat that sticks to cells. One place extra fat sticks is insulin receptors. This fat blocks our ability to use insulin. This is the beginning of type 2 diabetes and is called insulin resistance.

Obese people have higher levels of leptin because they don't respond to normal levels of leptin. Think of this as leptin insensitivity. An easy way to remember this is leptin resistance leads to overeating which makes extra calories turn to fat that stick to cells causing insulin resistance that then decreases adiponectin.

What where did that (adiponectin) come from? Well adiponectin lowers inflammation. High levels of leptin reduces levels of adiponectin, therefore inflammation markers rise in the body.

Think of it as leptin resistance goes hand in hand with insulin resistance leading to obesity and then diabetes and this leads to increases overall inflammation. (Leptin tells you that you are full.... insulin tells you that you are hungry).

Insulin helps push sugar into cells to be utilized as energy. When the insulin receptors are blocked your body has to over produce insulin in order to do what a healthy amount could do if you weren't overweight. The extra insulin in turn also makes you feel very hungry. So insulin resistant patients feel the need to eat extra calories that in turn MAKE YOU FAT.

Type 2, diabetes in turn reeks havoc upon your immune system and your ability to fight infections(COVID). It also is a leading factor associated with heart disease, kidney failure and blindness just for starters.

So obesity can lead to diabetes and so much more. Obesity causes your immune system to become overactive. I'll get to cytokines storm later but let's continue with obesity and the association with COVID.

Obese people suffer increased risk for complications from infections because obesity leads to an overactive immune system called inflammation. I mentioned this earlier. So obesity leads to inflammation and diabetes causes the same and that all leads to you immune system working in a dysfunctional manner. Your overactive immune system may not react normally to bacteria, fungi and viruses like it's supposed to(killing them). It can overreact and create the cytokines storm that destroys not only the invading organism but also the host(that's us).

FLU, COVID-19, SARS ETC. and OBESITY

A common clinical finding in all of the bad outcomes to every pandemic since the Spanish Flu and the current COVID-19 including the influenza that hit ten years ago is obesity! Two recent clinical reviews of over 7,000 patients combined showed obese patients with increased levels of inflammation which is correlated with increased heart disease and diabetes were far more likely to require hospitalization regardless of age! Physician's Weekly, April 14, 2020, Clinical Infectious Diseases, April 9, 2020 , Lancet, April 1, 2020 , Obesity, April 9, 2020). The vast majority of patients were elderly;however, for patients under 60 obesity doubles your chances of being hospitalized and requiring ventilator support. This finding is true for COVID, influenza, flu.... Obese people suffer increased risk for complications from infections because obesity leads to an overactive immune system called INFLAMMATION. This is where we started.

So if you want to reduce your personal chances of becoming severely ill during this or any other pandemic.....keep the weight off.

D. D. Jines. DMD,MD.

Adv Nutr. 2016;7:66-77

PLoS ONE, 2010; 5:e9694

Epidemiology, July 2015;26(4):580-589

Environ Toxicol Pharmacol, 2015;40(3):924-930

Nat Rev Immunol, 2011;11(2):85-97

IRON BUTT 5-3-2020

So the country is shut down and in parts locked down. What better way to express freedom and for me to CARPE DIEM!!! TWO IRON BUTT RIDES BACK TO BACK!!!

For those unfamiliar Iron Butt doesn't refer to that mean teacher or grandma. Iron Butt for the uninitiated is a 1000 mile ride in a day on a motorcycle. We've been doing them a few times a year for about two decades. This is the first with a drop of rain. St. Louis to Kansas City to enjoy the hospitality of Max and Deanna (Founder) and their lovely daughter and son in law Paul(Reguladores member)then at 4 AM a group(me, Bob,Jimmy,Max,Dick and Paul) of Reguladores rode down through Kansas, Oklahoma, Texas, New Mexico and ended up I Winslow Arizona by nightfall.

No rain just a guy passing a truck on a blind curve an a two lane. I was leading the group navigating so imagine semi truck directly to my left , I'm on crest heading down and BOZO whips out panics then proceeds to pass our group on our shoulder because he had to pass that truck. Inches...mere inches. Then a couple hours later were are again rolling and just moved to lane 2 as the slow lane was occupied by a white Chevy pickup pulling a trailer. Two angle iron loading ramps about 6 feet long but looked 20 ft easy especially when they fall off trailer into the path of a semi(solidly hit by semi) and again inches next to our group.

Our wives prayers worked.

I've posted and written about why riding with a club is fulfilling psychologically and spiritually and sharing this much fun is the great part of being in a group of like minded people. In this case cops.

SMALL WORLD. My former Chief and personal friend Dale Warke worked with and served in the military overseas 4 decades ago with a gentleman that later became a cop and now low and behold rides motorcycles and is in the same club. Down in Texas. My friend Mike who served with me on the Police Dept. in Lebanon moved in the early 2000's and became a police chief in Santa Rosa New Mexico. He later became the county Sheriff in that county and now he will soon be a Charter Member and President if his own chapter of Reguladores. Our group stopped into Mike's new Microbrewery and bar that's under construction, since we were in the neighborhood.

IRON BUTT II FOR THE FIRST WEEKEND OF MAY 2020. RANDOM THOUGHTS.....

RAGIN CAJUN 2020
Each May first for a decade we've loaded up the bike and headed to Lafayette Louisiana for the **REGULADORES LEMC** Super Party called RAGIN CAJUN. COVID reared its ugliness and we are doing our version of social distancing by riding a little under 3000

miles doing two Iron Butt Rides(1000 miles or more in 24 hours... my record is 1680 in 30 hours).

COVID, Trump derangement syndrome, crashing economy, personal struggles, strife, loss of Rights.....all seem to disappear when we are with kindred souls and freedom loving patriots. The miles didn't matter as all of that was replaced with scenic vistas and remarkable views of nature's beauty combined with the moving of our collective souls while perched upon our iron horses.....alright the Harley riders were saddled upon iron horses while I was safely ensconced (more like wearing) becoming one with my aluminum and carbon fiber and plastic Can Am. Hey you all have to admit it gets the job done especially from a standing stop!

REGULADORES LEMC RECRUITING EFFORT

We took the opportunity to meet and greet my friend and former fellow Lebanon Police Officer Mike Chavez. He left Illinois and became Chief of Police in Santa Rosa before becoming the county Sheriff of same. He will be starting a brand new chapter of Reguladores soon and we will definitely be headed there as he is also building a brand new microbrewery and restaurant! Talk about great club meeting place!

PAIN IN THE NECK

As you all know I have ALS. It weakens muscles and if you work out it kills the muscles even faster. Many times you'll see an ALS patient in a wheelchair with their head propped up or strapped to a headrest because the neck muscles are no longer able to support the head upright. Neck pain occurs as the head acts like a dead weight causing pressure to build upon nerves. For the last seven years I've gone to my neurologist Dr. Worth for in office therapy and as soon as the IRON BUTT ride was over and a shower and lunch Darla dropped me off for a few days of relief.

THANKFULNESS

Thank you all for riding with me this weekend and those that rode over from Louisiana. During all of this weekend's fun hundreds died from hunger, heart disease, violence, world strife, pestilence,.....just kidding they all died of COVID. Seriously we made a choice to leave all of that in the rear view mirrors and enjoy the company of people who are of like mind and spirit.

Our Gremlin Bells worked overtime! Steel ramps falling off a trailer in front of us was just one event...then the guy passing oncoming semi truck on a blind hill then veering onto our shoulder missing us by meer inches was another and then there was the lady that wanted her Uhaul truck to occupy the space already occupied by Bob and his Ultra while going 80 mph. (It's all good Bob has hit guard rails much tougher that the sides of that truck).

COURAGE

I witnessed Founder Max straighten out a car load of twenty somethings in the gas pump line when they cut in line and bumped his foot peg. Many demure to flagrant rude behavior; however, Max made me remember a scene from Lonesome Dove about rude behavior and the fact Capt. McCall didn't tolerate it. He thinks it's nothing but I can tell you many modern men demure against greater odds so when I see a man stand his ground it gets me in the feels.

REGULADORES LEMC is a group of individuals many of whom have lived lives like the ones Hollywood likes to use for their stories.

At least one has been immortalized by his own actions but also by Hollywood in film. When these individuals become a group with a single purpose it's an opportunity to make the world better and it is because of their works. Being surrounded even for a short time by you all makes all the rest bearable. RFFR!

PS.....

The song lyric that Jackson Browne and Glenn Frey wrote,"Take it Easy" is about handling life's tough moments in stride. That's what we did!!!

MOTHER'S DAY 2020

Strength, character, love, honor, dignity, perseverance are just a few of the attributes I use to describe my mother. She is the one that taught me if I wanted self esteem I'd better earn it. She taught me if I wanted dignity and respect I'd better earn it. If I wanted to act like any fool on Maury or Jerry Springer I'd never have either. My mother taught me that I could be anything I wanted even when others discouraged my dreams. My mother was my father's rock and is the glue that holds this family together. We thank her today and honor her constant loyalty and love. She is a typical Asian tiger mom who demands more than most and expects even more. I remember her telling me and my brothers," if you use drugs...lie, cheat, steal...or in anyway dishonor your family, your name or me and dad...kill yourself". She meant it. I love my mom.

Chisi

And now to all the other mothers in my life including..... TO: Darla Porter-Jines, Laura Ann Polito, Sophia Jines, Alana Kratochwil, Karlie Melton, Carly Melton, Sue Hughes- Jines , Marta Ince Jines,

Hannah Witt , Amanda Mattler, Judy Porter and My Mom and all the other Moms our there in my family , friends and world.

SUBJ: MOTHERS DAY

First let me express my sincere gratitude for your selfless sacrifice made daily. You all are examples of GOD'S love and I'm forever and daily reminded of that gift through your actions, words and example.

When one talks of the labor of love all I need do is witness how you care for your children, keep your homes, work outside to help make ends meet or sacrifice your own material wants for your families.

I recently read a story about a former First Lady who felt having children was a burden that ruined her career. I am so proud and thankful that you chose to give your life's focus to all of us, without one hint that I or we were a burden.

I am so proud I know you and to love each and every one of you. Thank you.

Denzel.

THE END OF THIS BOOK FOR NOW!

Thanking Staff

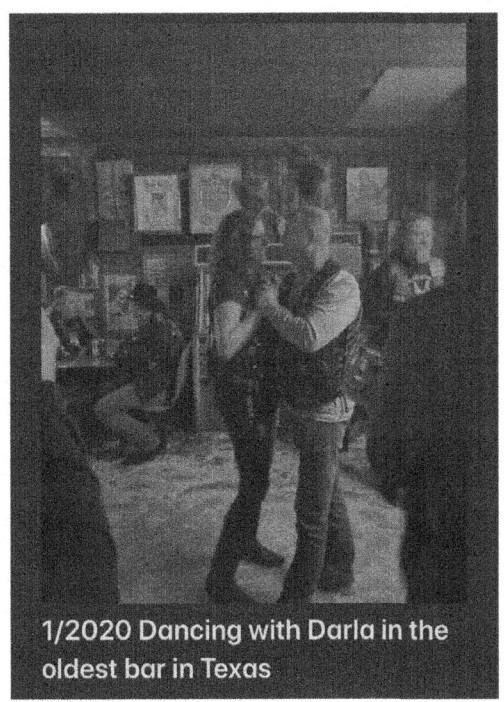

1/2020 Dancing with Darla in the oldest bar in Texas

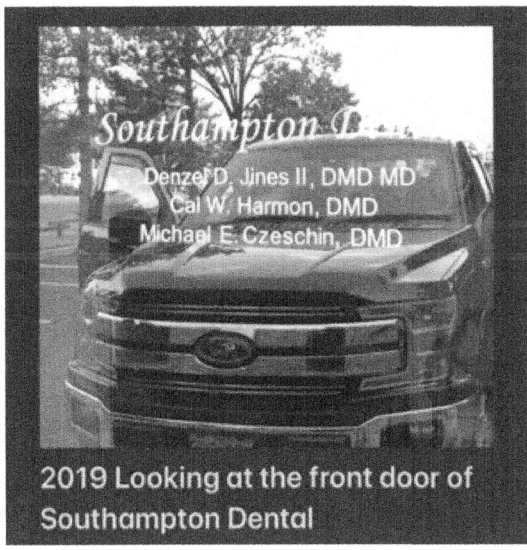

2019 Looking at the front door of Southampton Dental

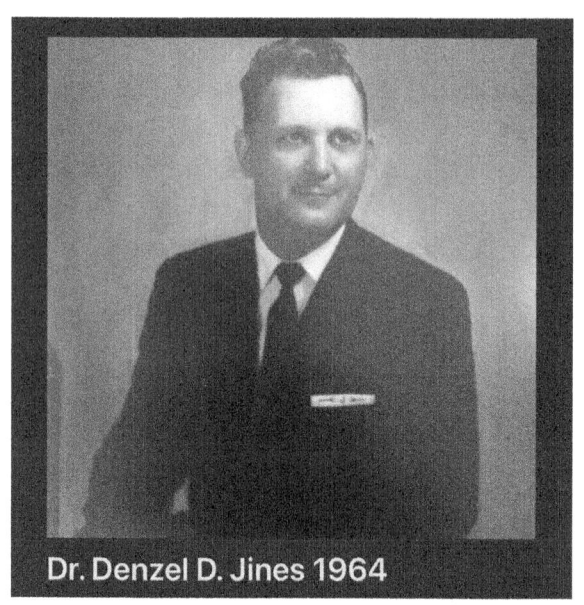

Dr. Denzel D. Jines 1964

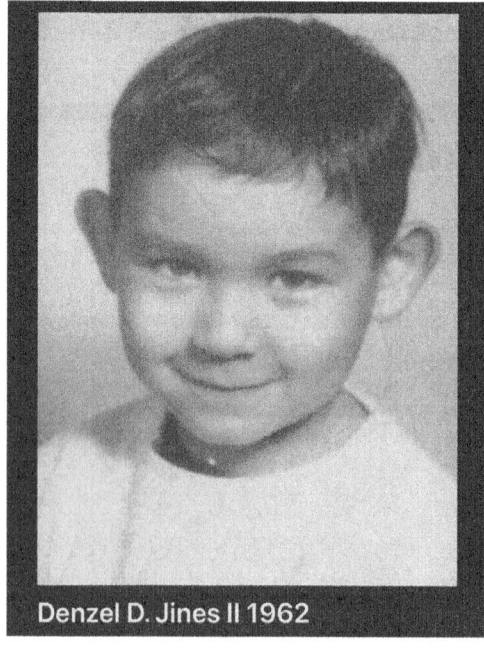

Denzel D. Jines II 1962

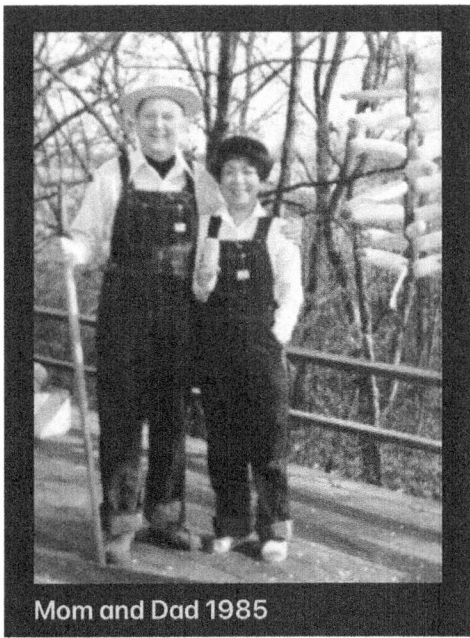

Mom and Dad 1985

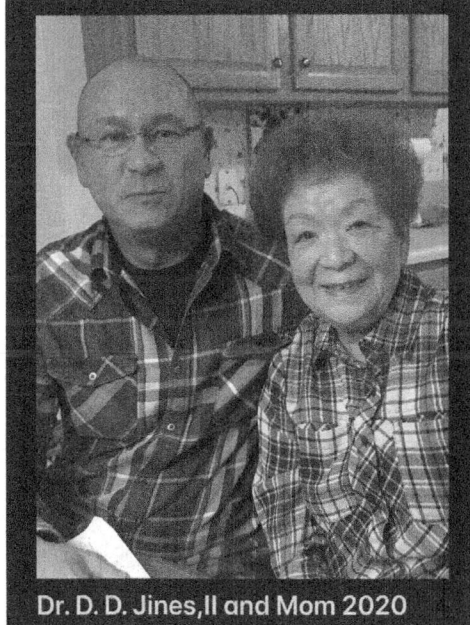

Dr. D. D. Jines,II and Mom 2020

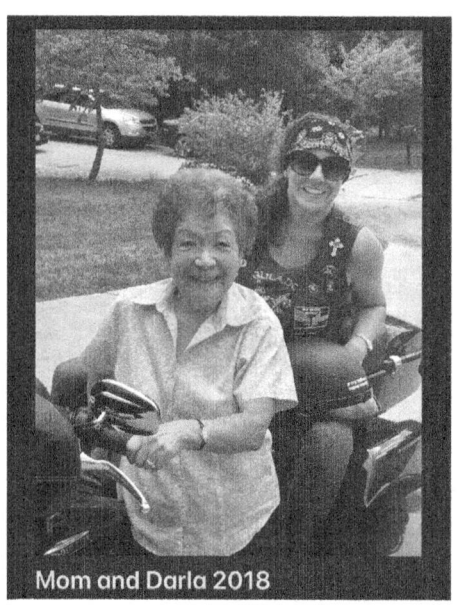

Mom and Darla 2018

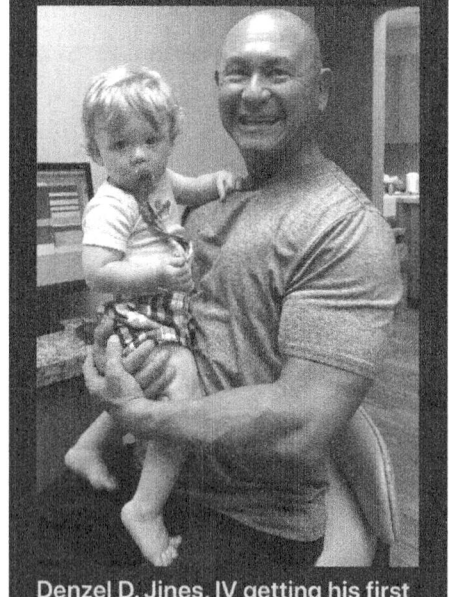

Denzel D. Jines, IV getting his first dental exam from grandpa Denzel II , 2016

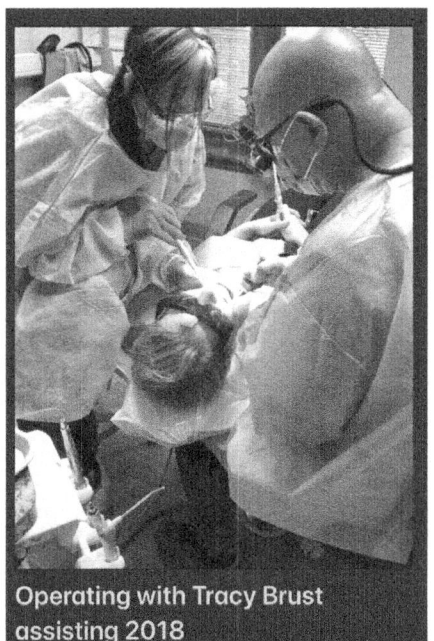

Operating with Tracy Brust assisting 2018

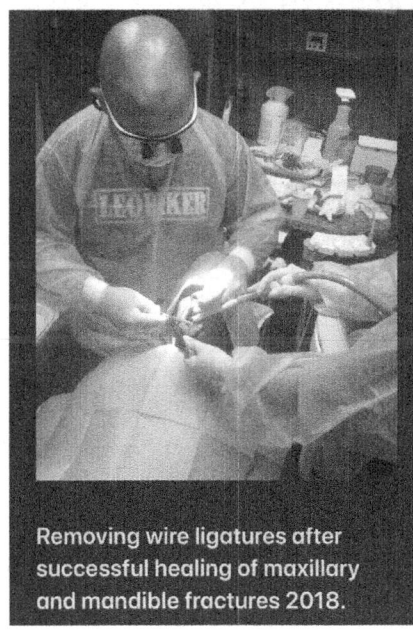

Removing wire ligatures after successful healing of maxillary and mandible fractures 2018.

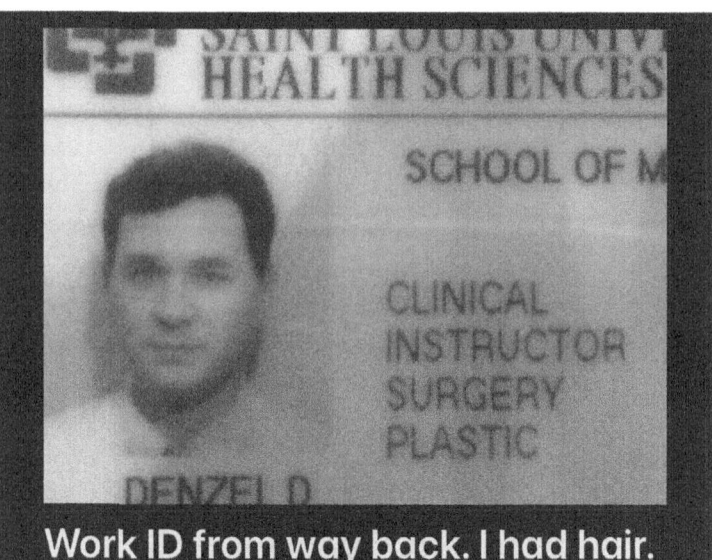

Work ID from way back. I had hair.

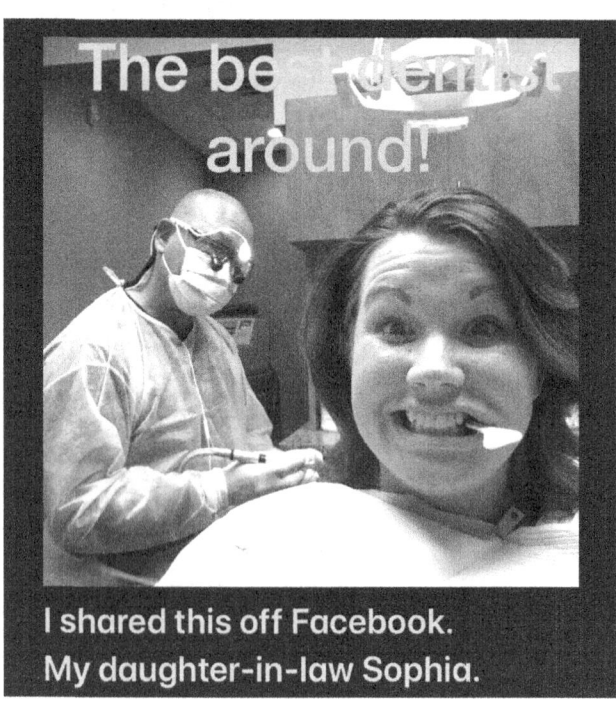

I shared this off Facebook.
My daughter-in-law Sophia.

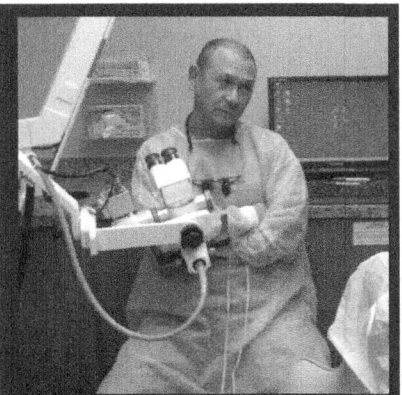

That face you make when someone is about to tell you all those cavities were because weak teeth just run in the family and have nothing to do with the 10 Mountain Dews, 4 bags of skittles and two daily hits if Meth.

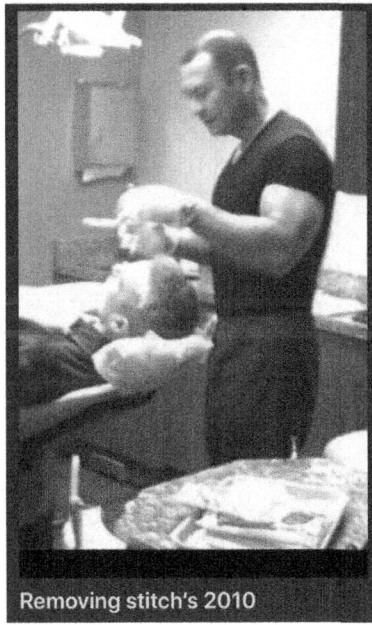

Removing stitch's 2010

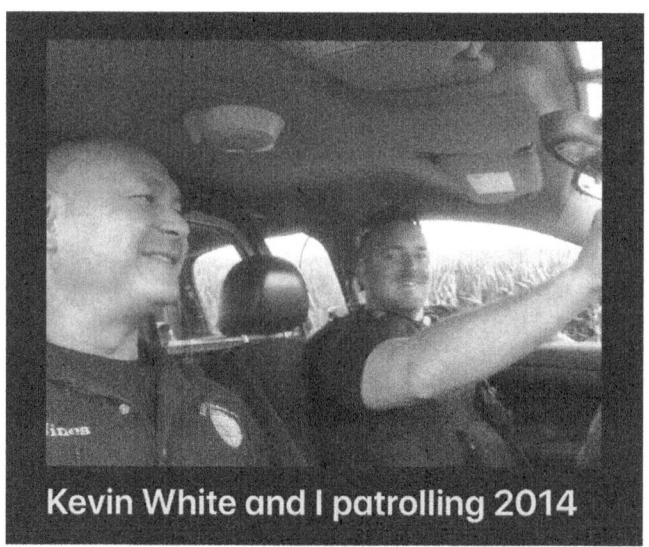

Kevin White and I patrolling 2014

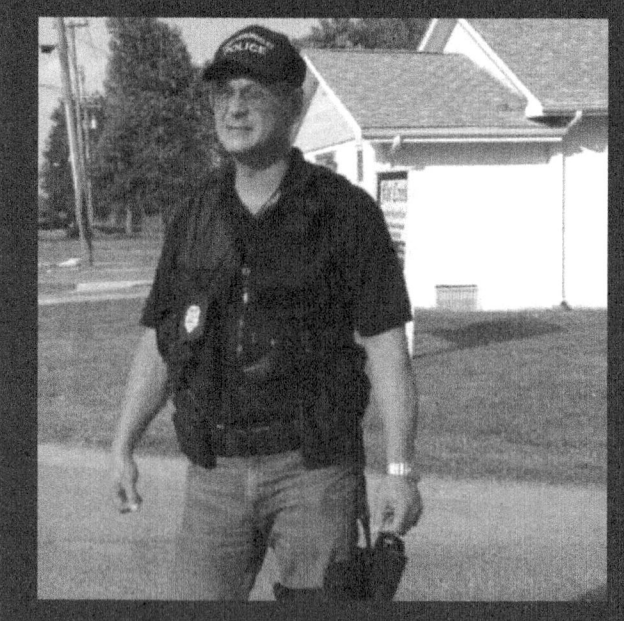

High Noon Safety and DUI
Checkpoint 2010

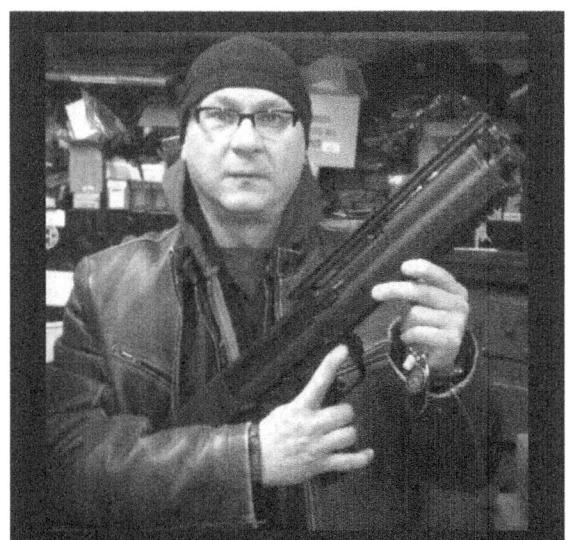

Being an Illinois State Certified Police Firearms Instructor had the advantage of getting to see the newest technology.

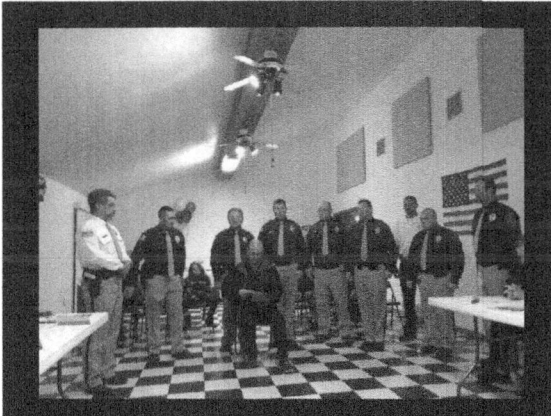

Retirement Orders Received From Chief Michael Dennis and Mayor Herbert Simmons 2016.

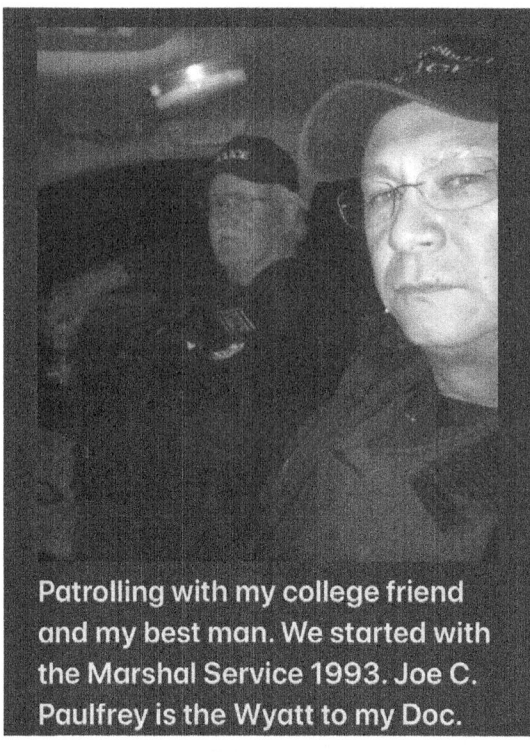

Patrolling with my college friend and my best man. We started with the Marshal Service 1993. Joe C. Paulfrey is the Wyatt to my Doc.

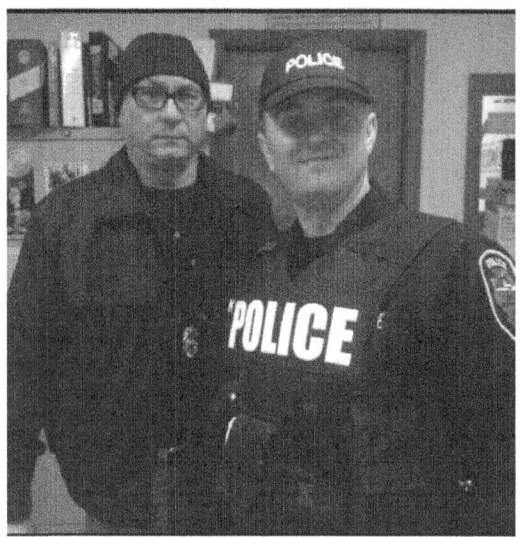

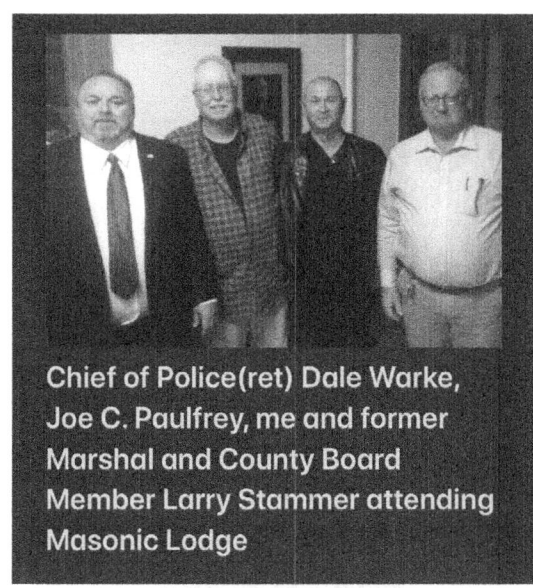

Chief of Police(ret) Dale Warke, Joe C. Paulfrey, me and former Marshal and County Board Member Larry Stammer attending Masonic Lodge

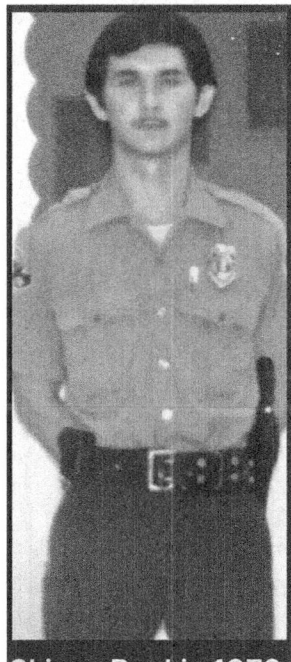

Skinny Rookie 1979

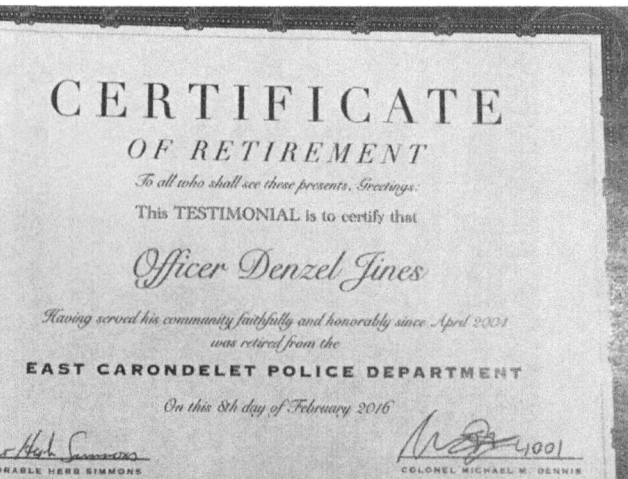

CERTIFICATE

OF RETIREMENT

To all who shall see these presents, Greetings:

This TESTIMONIAL is to certify that

Officer Denzel Jines

Having served his community faithfully and honorably since April 2001
was retired from the

EAST CARONDELET POLICE DEPARTMENT

On this 8th day of February 2016

HONORABLE HERB SIMMONS
MAYOR

COLONEL MICHAEL M. DENNIS
CHIEF OF POLICE

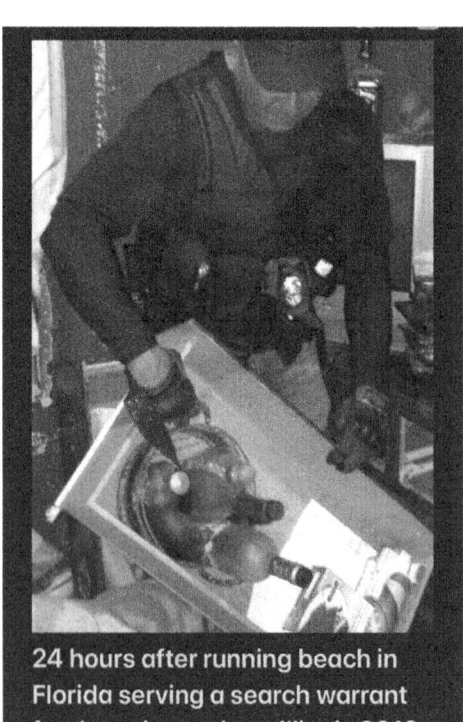

24 hours after running beach in Florida serving a search warrant for drugs in southern Illinois 2012

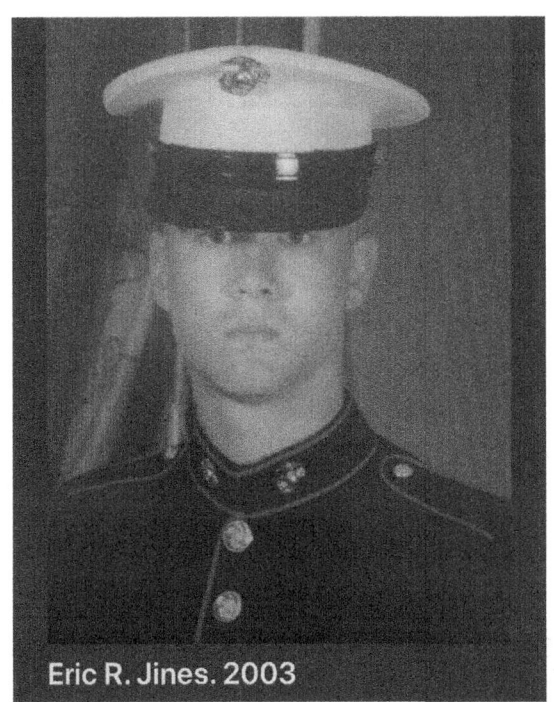

Eric R. Jines. 2003

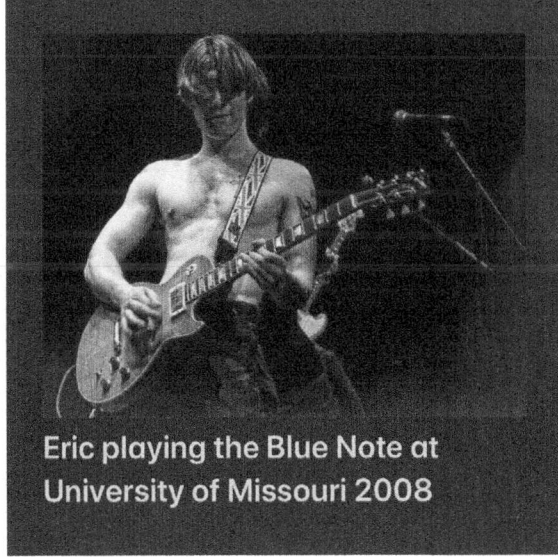

Eric playing the Blue Note at
University of Missouri 2008

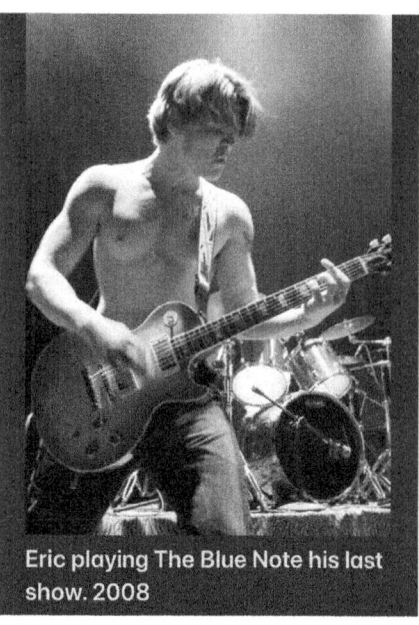

Eric playing The Blue Note his last show. 2008

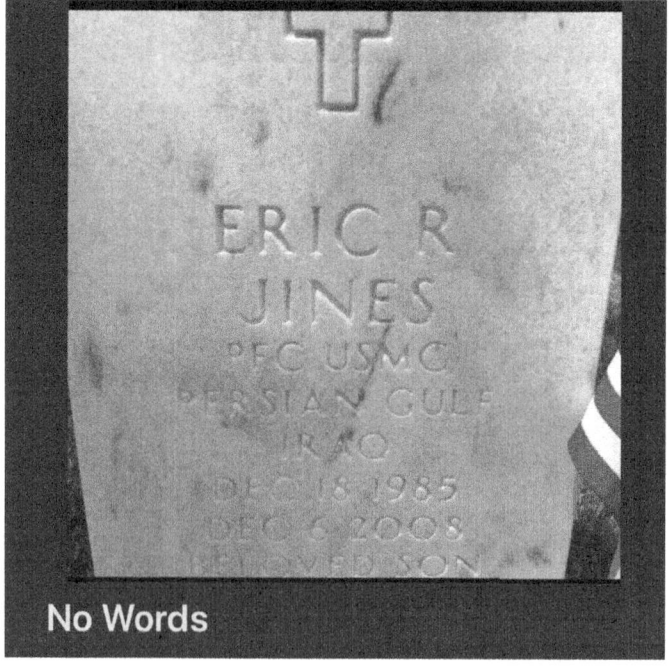

No Words

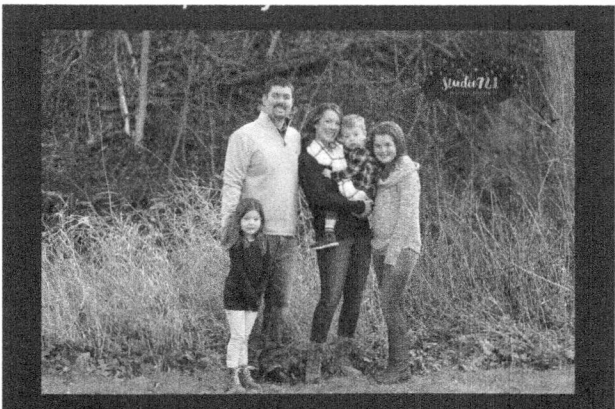

Denzel, Sophia, little Dean with big sister Addysen and middle sister Bristol

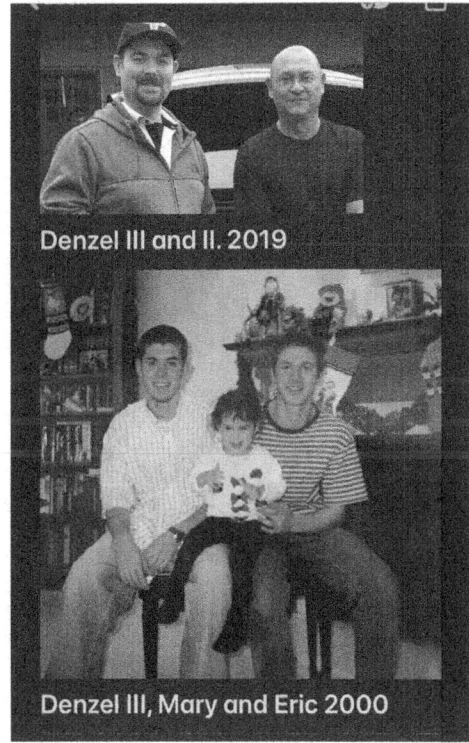

Denzel III and II. 2019

Denzel III, Mary and Eric 2000

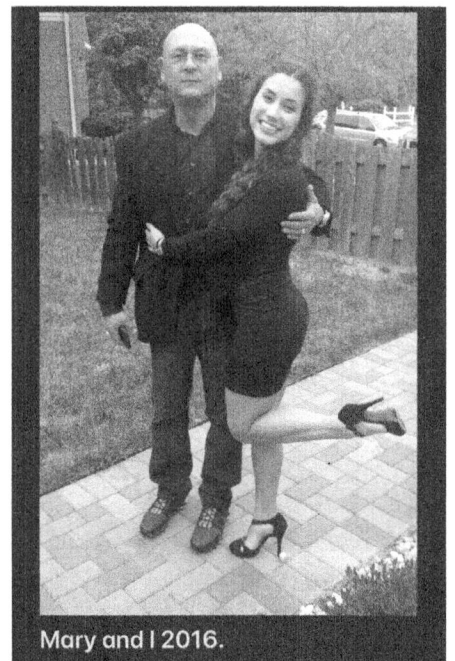

Mary and I 2016.

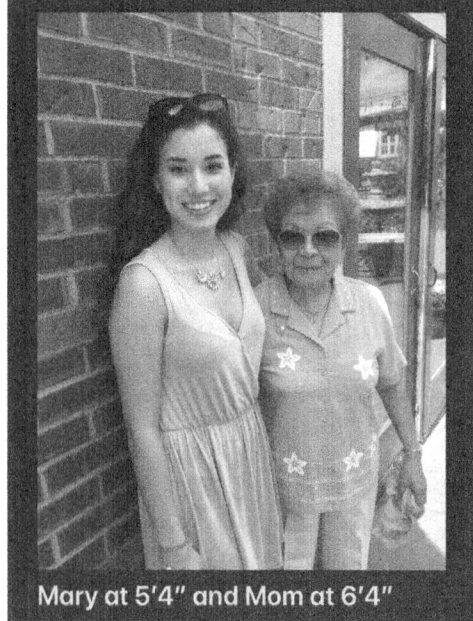

Mary at 5'4" and Mom at 6'4"

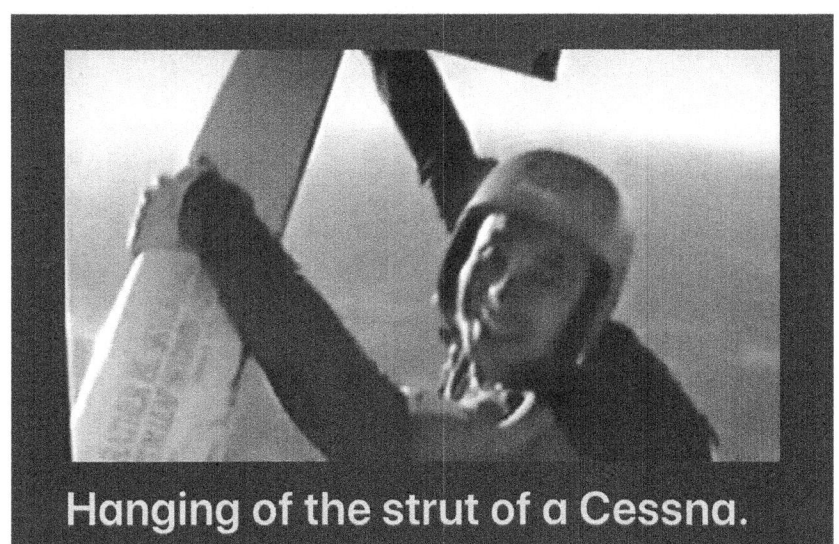

Hanging of the strut of a Cessna.

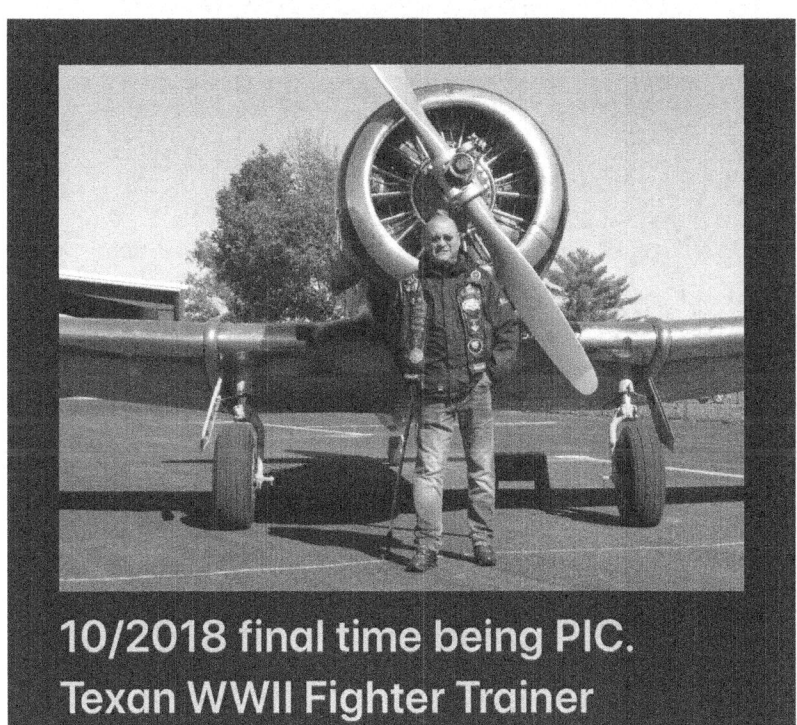

10/2018 final time being PIC.
Texan WWII Fighter Trainer

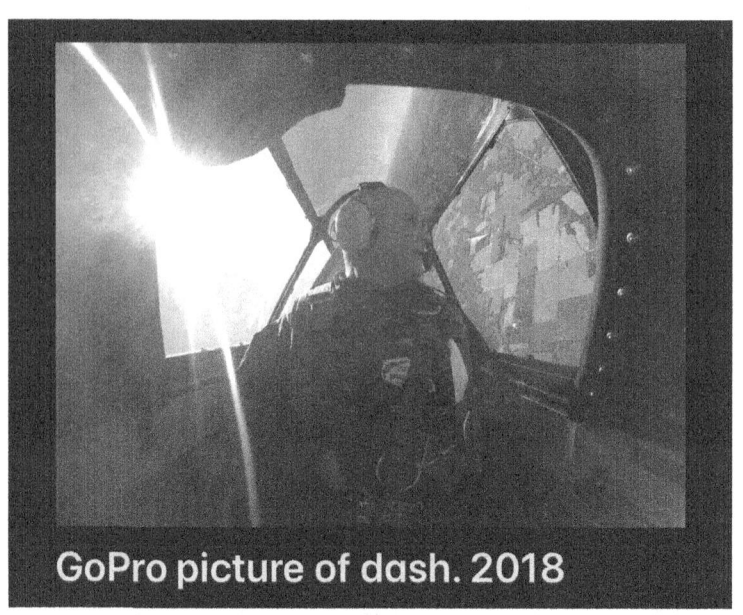

GoPro picture of dash. 2018

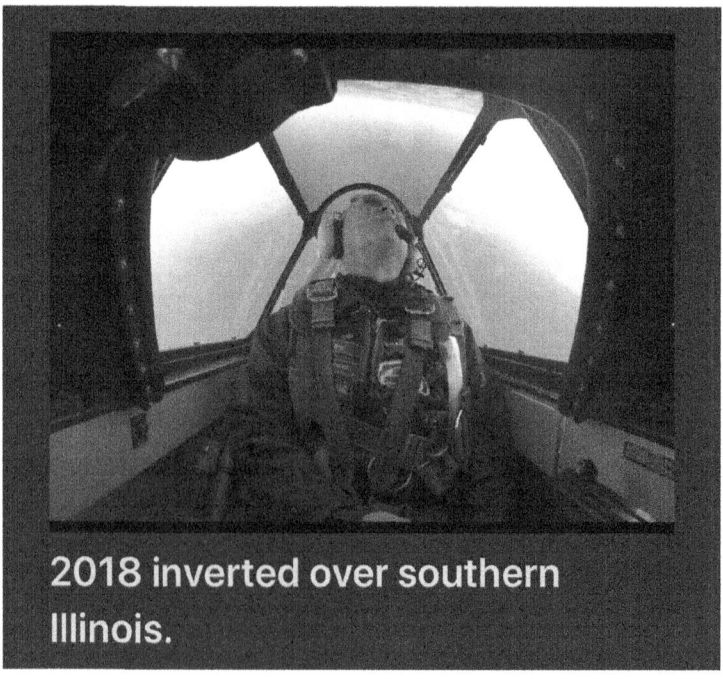

2018 inverted over southern Illinois.

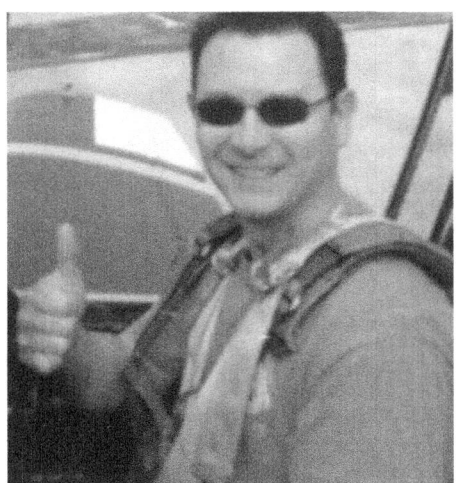

PIC in a Texan a WWII advanced fighter trainer...20 years earlier than my last time flying one of these(10-21-2018)

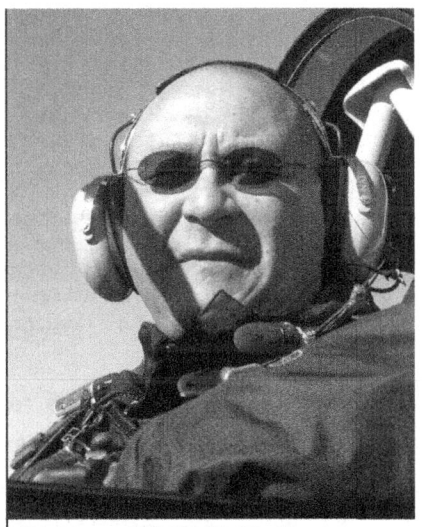

Front seat PIC 10-21-18...Texan N97VR built 1942 was an advanced fighter trainer and this was my second time to fly this particular model.

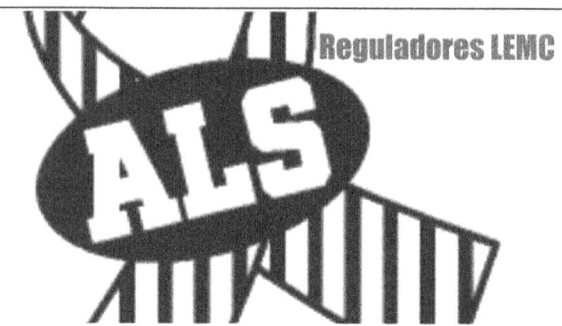

Reguladores LEMC

Fundraiser for The ALS Association - St. Louis Regional Chapter by Vanessa Peterson • ⊕ Public

About

In honor of those who have lost the battle with ALS and those who continue to fight, the Reguladores LEMC invite you to contibute to The ALS Association - St. Louis Regional Chapter. Your contribution will make an impact, whether you donate $5 or $500. Every little bit helps. Thank you for your support. We've included information about The ALS Association - St. Louis Regional Chapter below.

Our mission is to discover treatments and a cure for ALS, and to serve, advocate for, and empower people affected by ALS to live their lives to the fullest.

 Vanessa Peterson • September 15, 2018

Reguladores LEMC Sister Vanessa Peterson posted this on Facebook during the build up to the "ARREST ALS "event 10/18

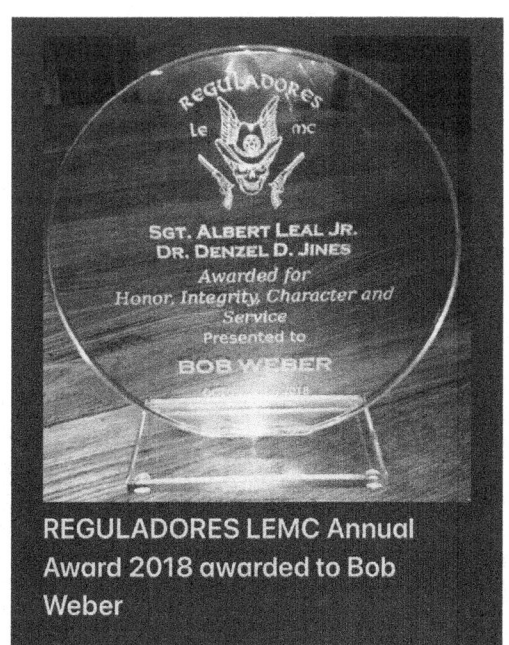

REGULADORES LEMC Annual
Award 2018 awarded to Bob
Weber

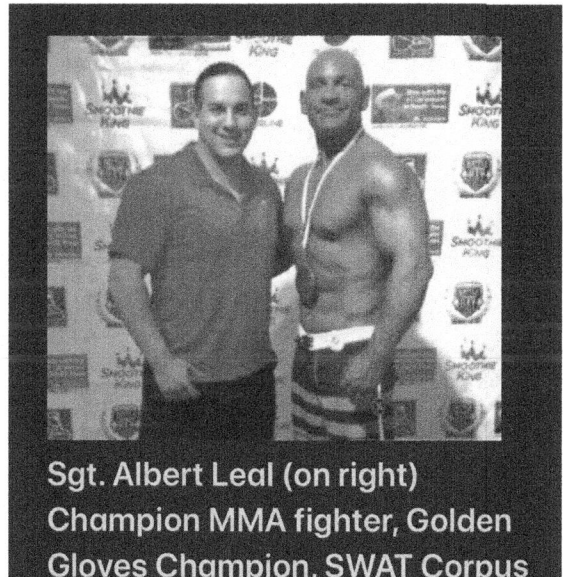

Sgt. Albert Leal (on right)
Champion MMA fighter, Golden
Gloves Champion, SWAT Corpus
Christy PD.

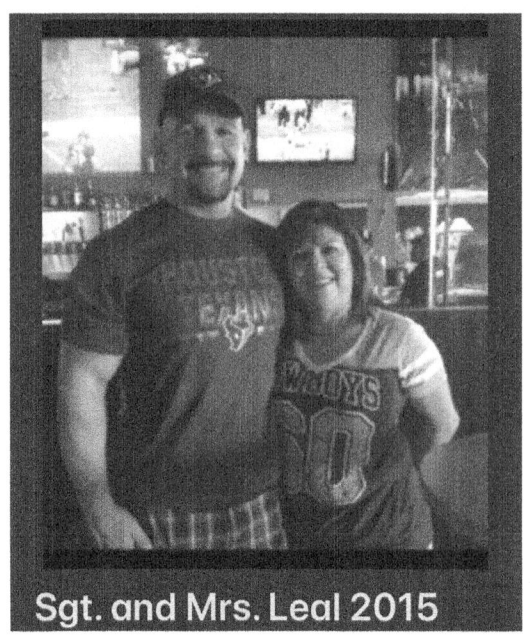

Sgt. and Mrs. Leal 2015

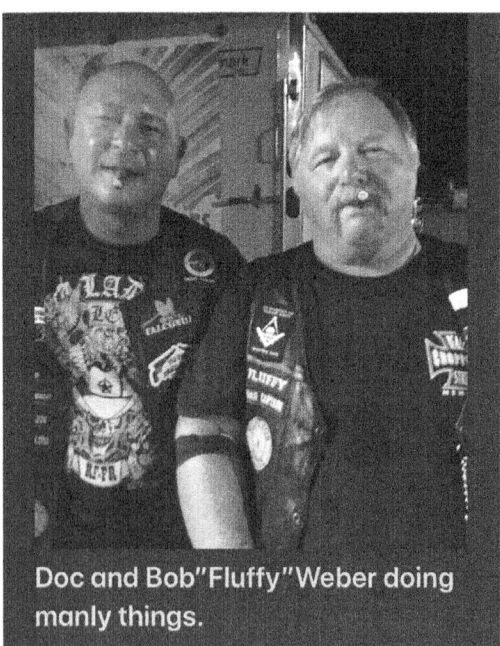

Doc and Bob"Fluffy"Weber doing manly things.

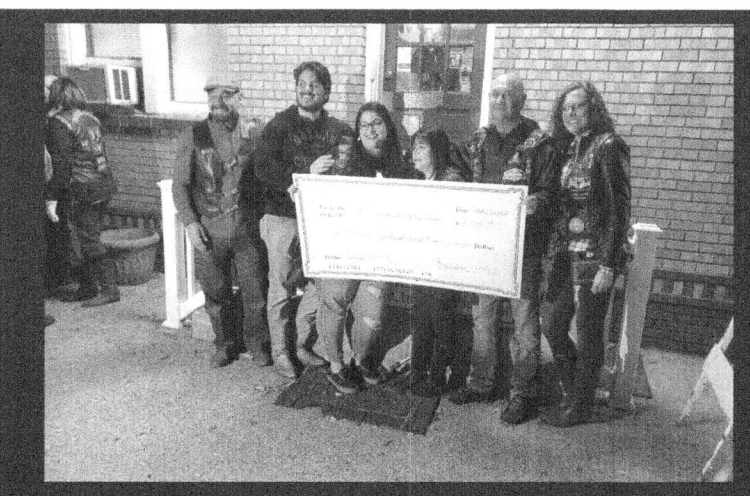

Check presentation to ALS Association of St. Louis from Reguladores LEMC 2018

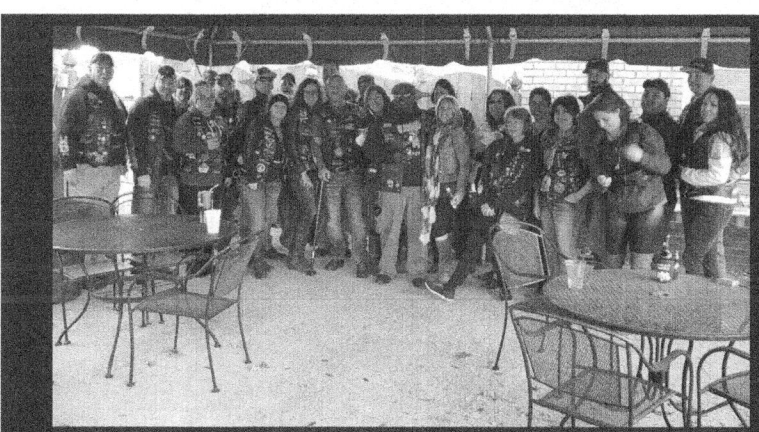

Reguladores LEMC at Arrest ALS 2018 in Southern Illinois.

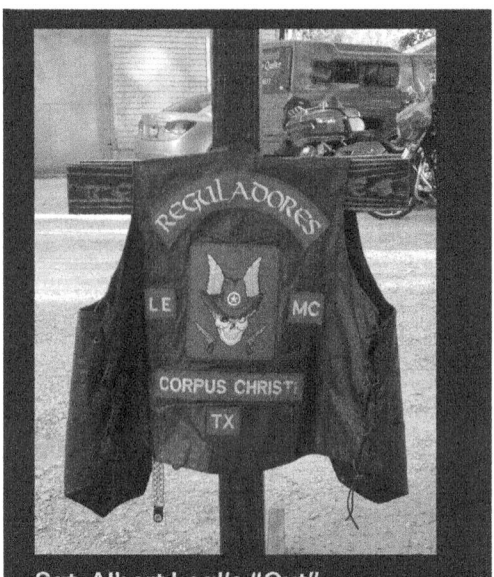

Sgt. Albert Leal's "Cut".

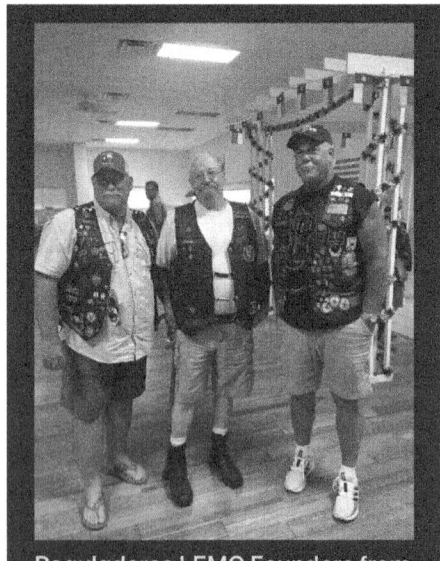

Reguladores LEMC Founders from left:Ron Zirbes,Curtis Shelton,Richard Maxwell

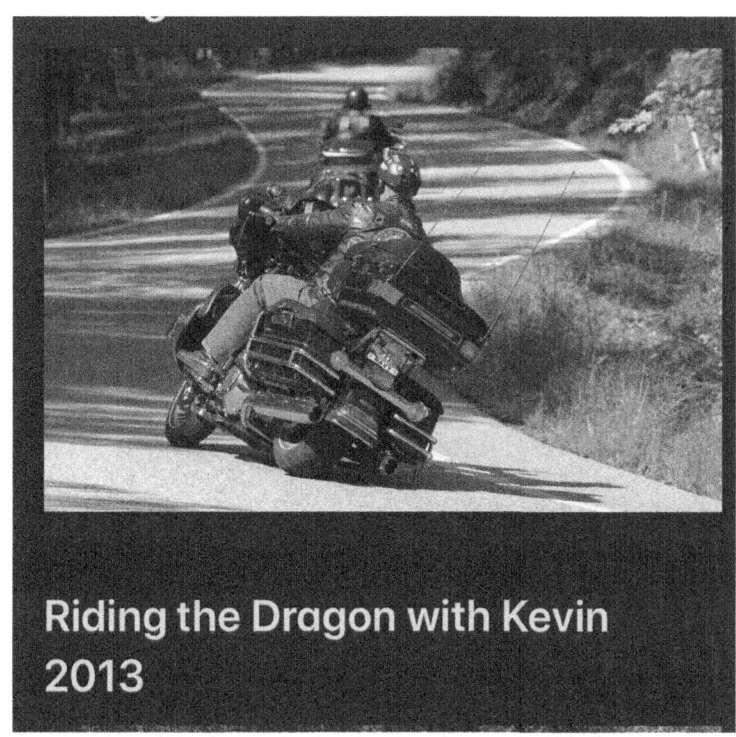

Riding the Dragon with Kevin 2013

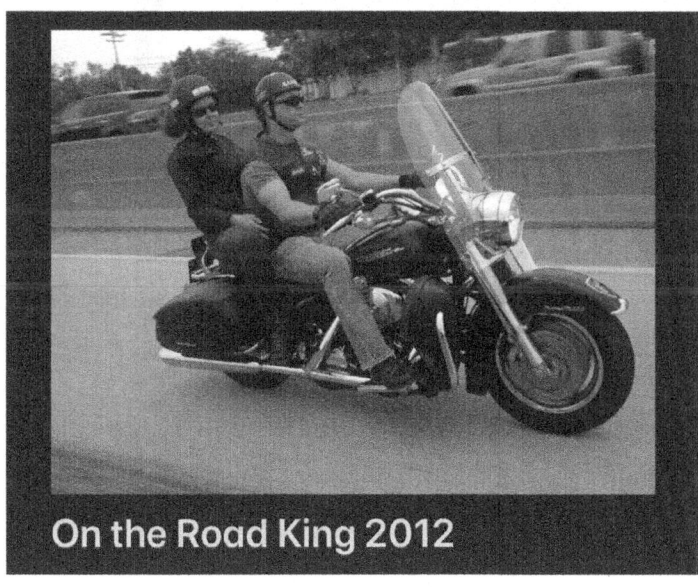

On the Road King 2012

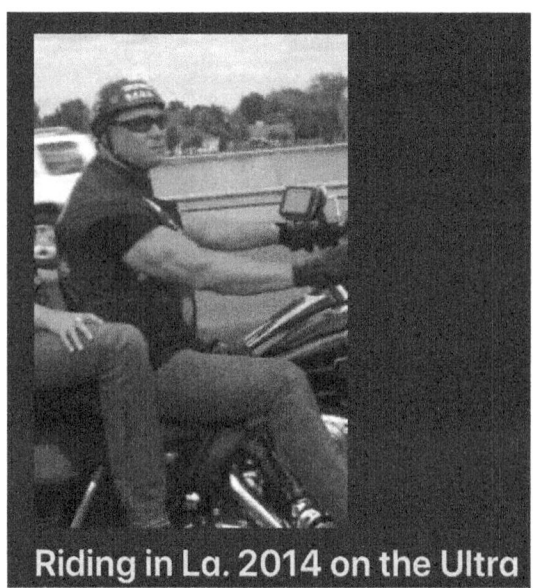

Riding in La. 2014 on the Ultra

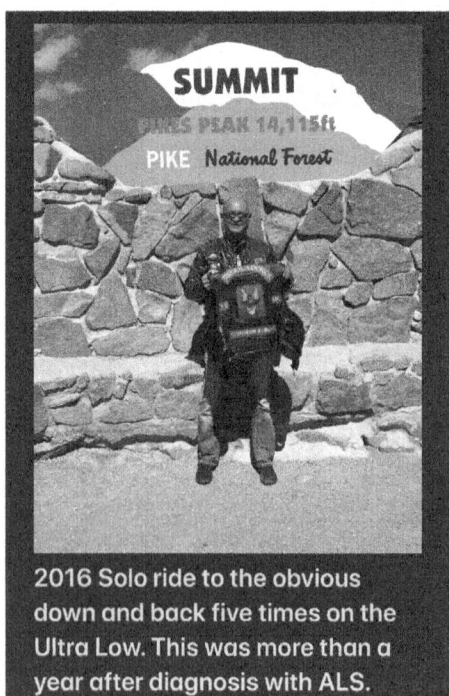

SUMMIT

PIKES PEAK 14,115ft

PIKE *National Forest*

2016 Solo ride to the obvious
down and back five times on the
Ultra Low. This was more than a
year after diagnosis with ALS.

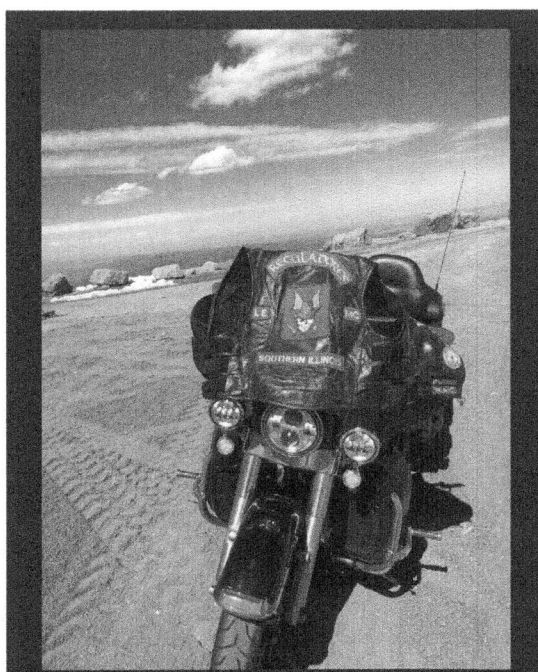

Riding Pike's Peak 2016.

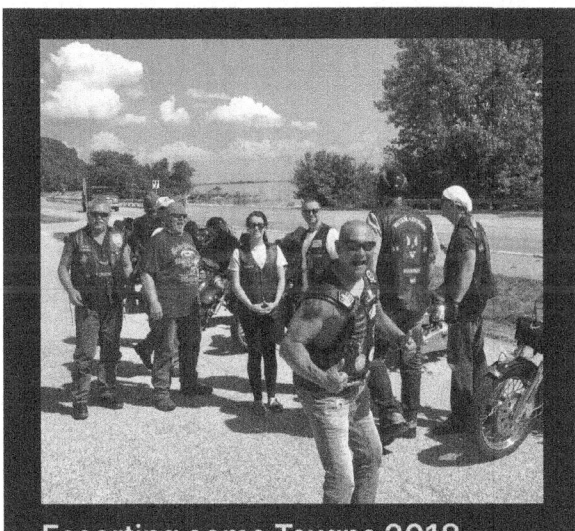

Escorting some Texans 2018

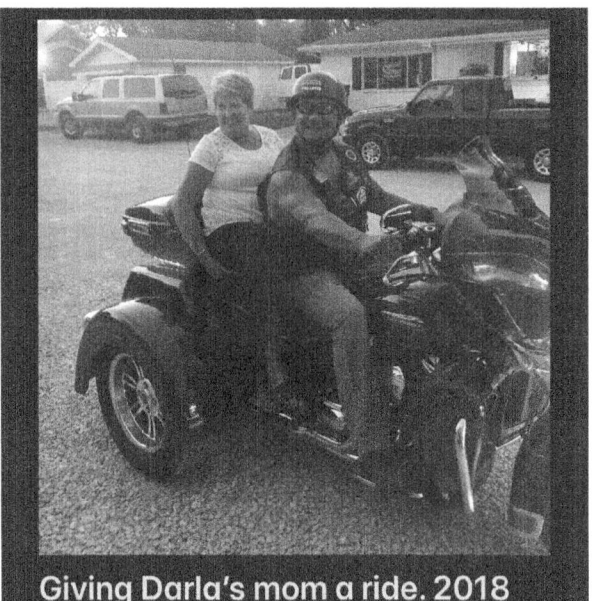

Giving Darla's mom a ride. 2018

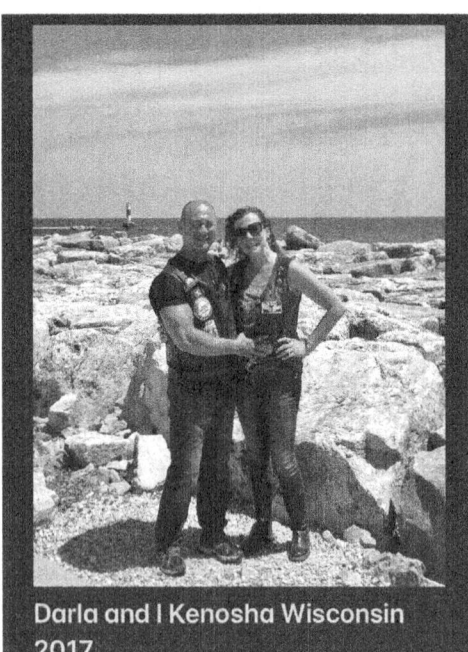

Darla and I Kenosha Wisconsin 2017

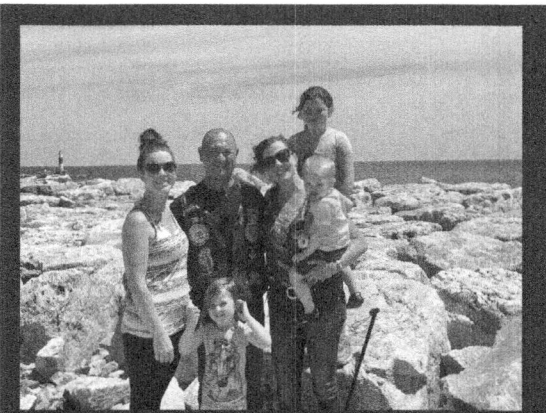

Sophia Jines and Bristol, Addy, Dean with Darla and me in Kenosha 2018.

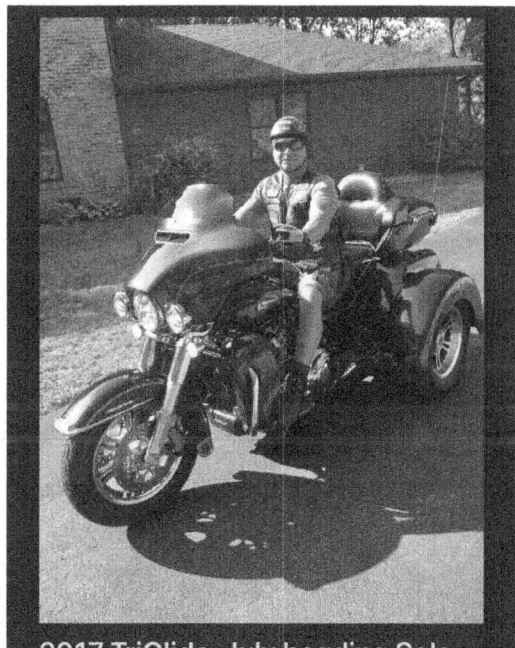

2017 TriGlide. July heading Solo to Texas Nationals.

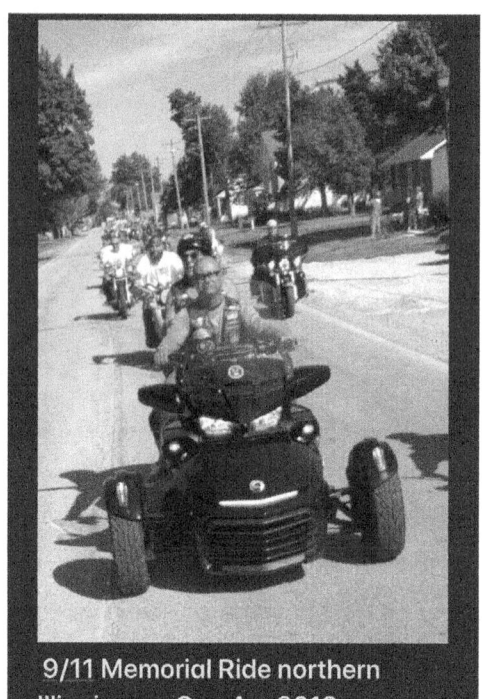

9/11 Memorial Ride northern Illinois on a Can Am 2019

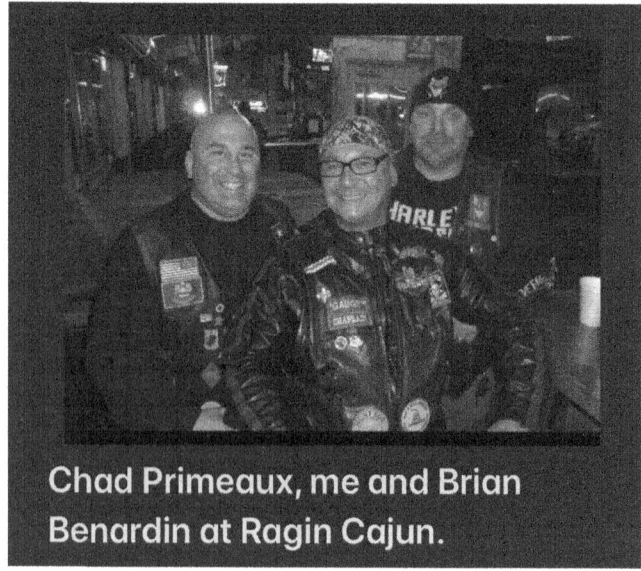

Chad Primeaux, me and Brian Benardin at Ragin Cajun.

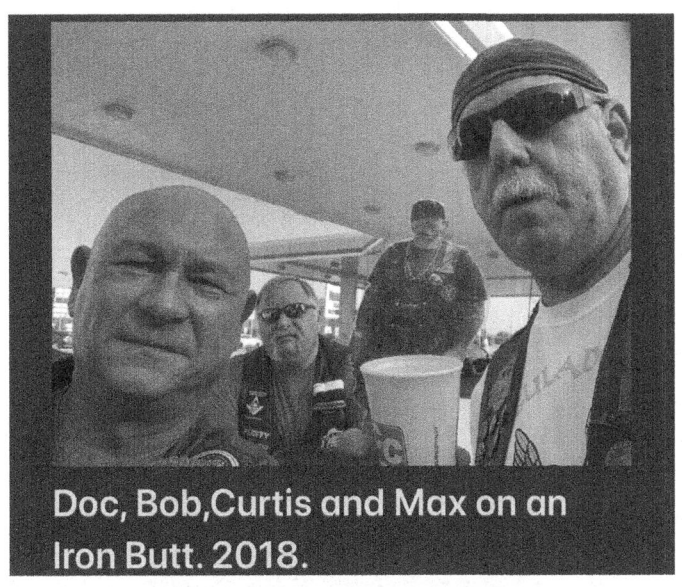

Doc, Bob,Curtis and Max on an Iron Butt. 2018.

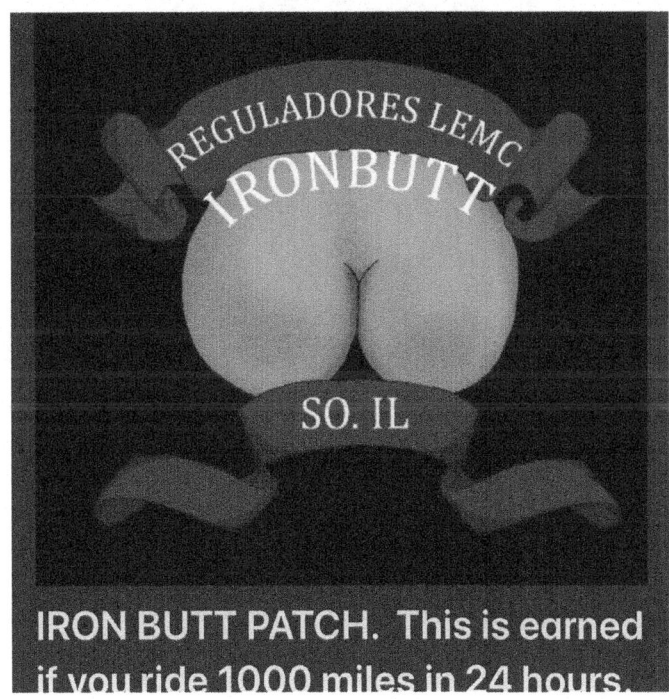

IRON BUTT PATCH. This is earned if you ride 1000 miles in 24 hours.

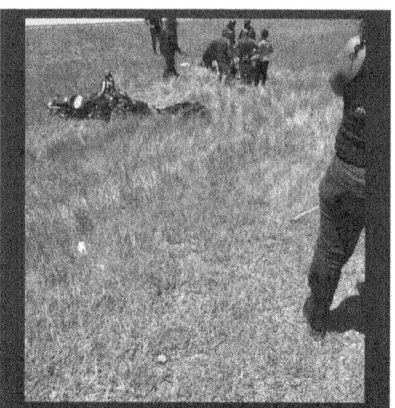

Treating a roadside casualty in Tennessee 2018. I wrote a clinical post about being prepared for emergencies not just in the clinic. I was the only doctor for fifteen minutes. It took 45 minutes for a Life Flight helicopter to get there.

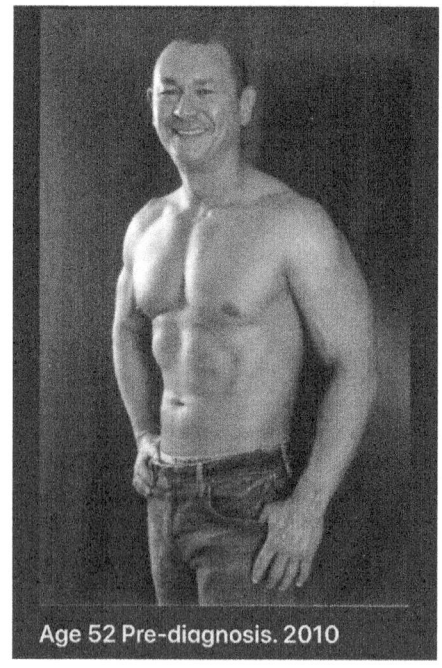

Age 52 Pre-diagnosis. 2010

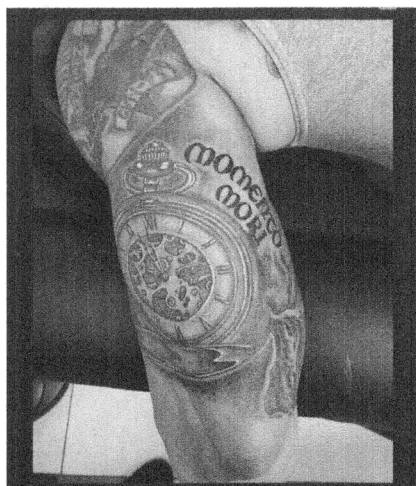

The Watch measures our most precious asset. The Memento Mori reminds us we all die. The ship above is my ship USS THEODORE ROOSEVELT.

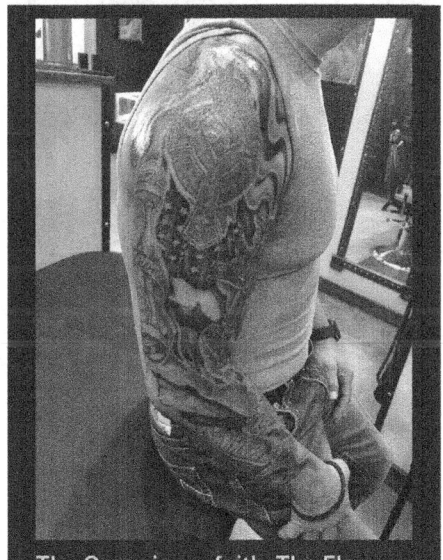

The Cross is my faith. The Flag underneath my country.

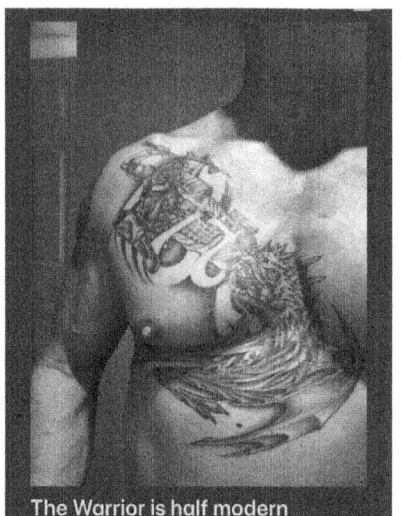

The Warrior is half modern operator. The other half is a salute to my ancestors and is a traditional Samurai.

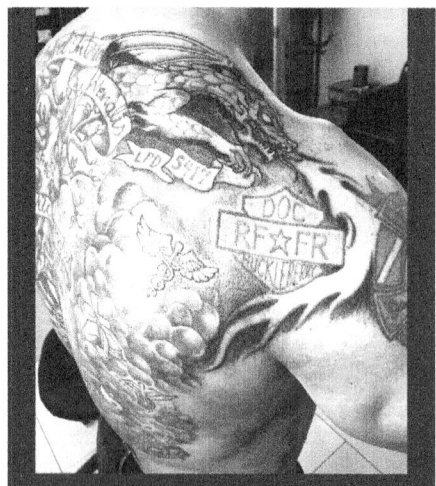

The Japanese Dragon my badge number and Road Name. The Medical and Dental Caduceus and a Bible representing my Ordination.

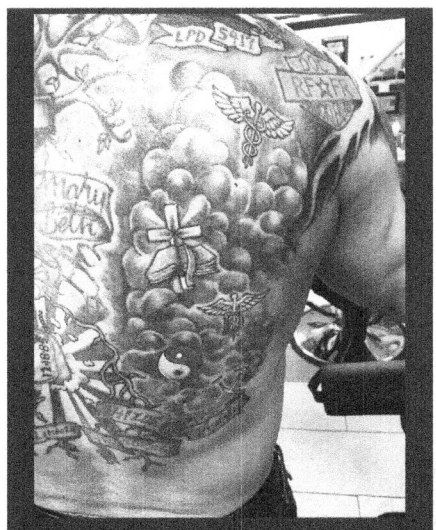

View of right back. The Ying Yang is a symbol of one of my martial arts black belts.

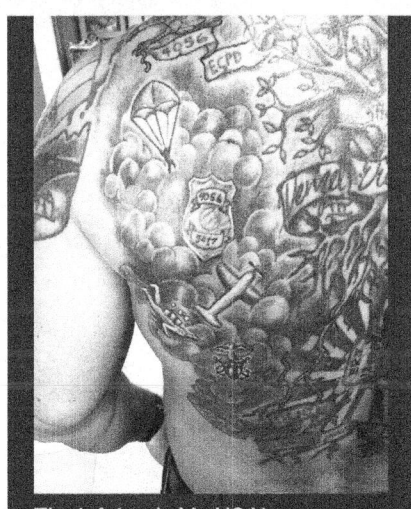

The left back. My US Navy Officers Insignia, the Plane and Divers represent my pilots's, skydiving, and SCUBA licenses.

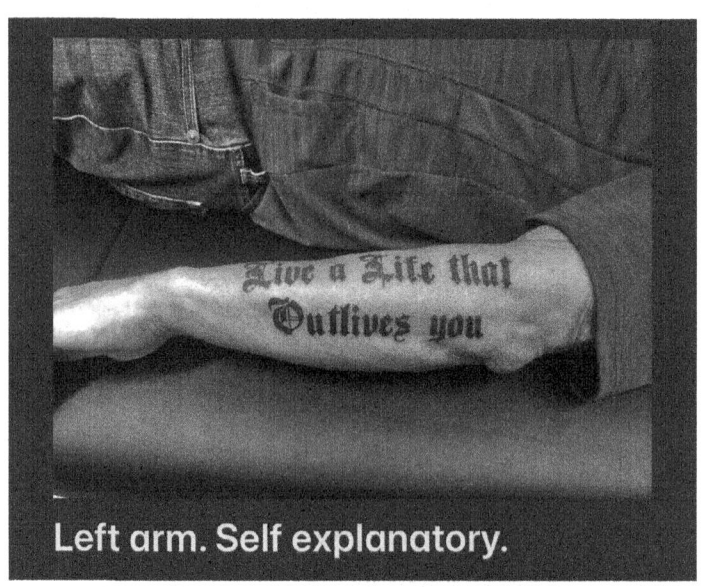

Left arm. Self explanatory.

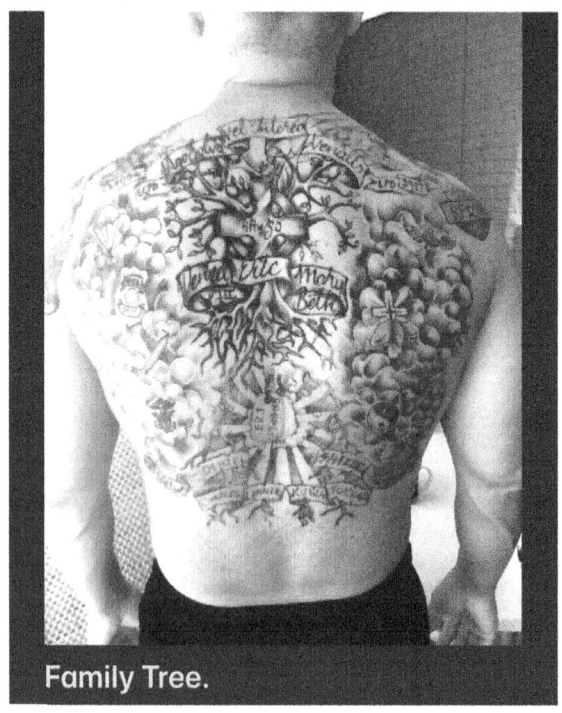

Family Tree.

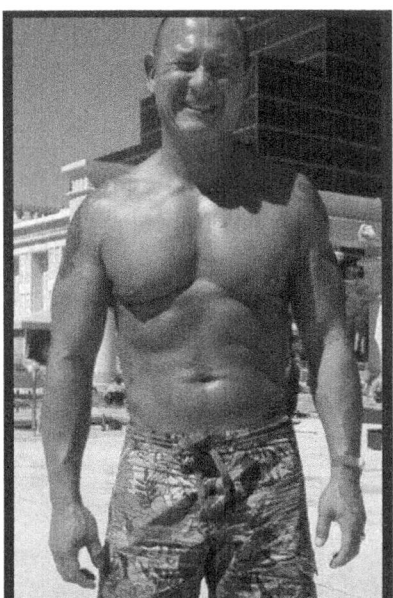

55 years old 2013 cropping out shrinking legs.

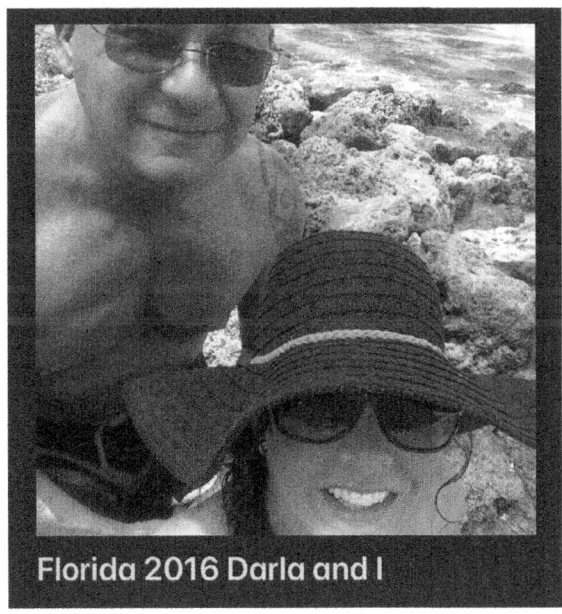

Florida 2016 Darla and I

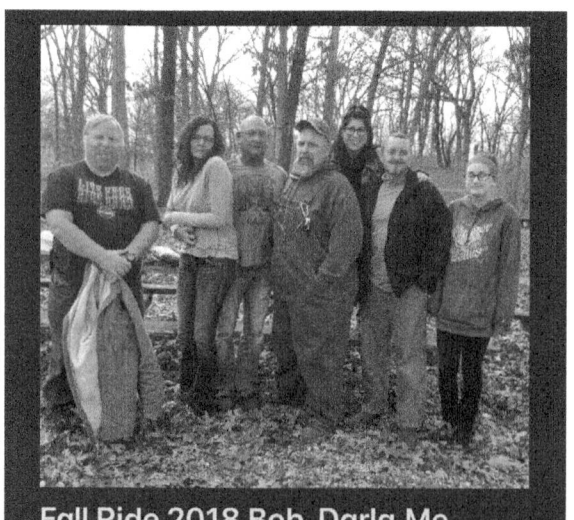

Fall Ride 2018 Bob, Darla,Me,
Brian, Vanessa, Kevin and Macy

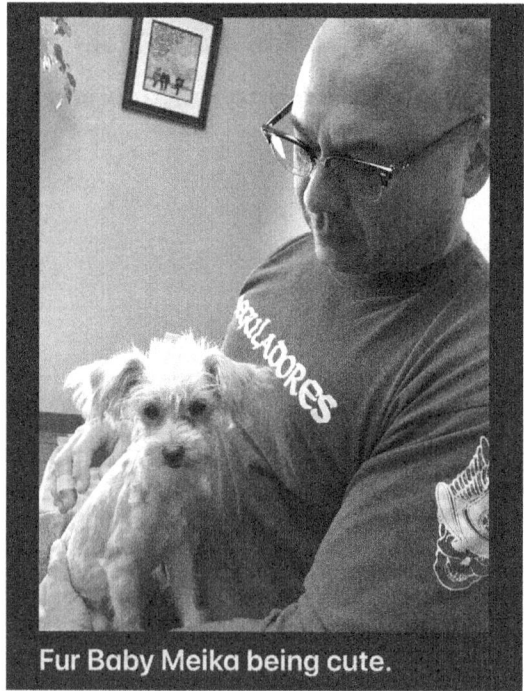

Fur Baby Meika being cute.

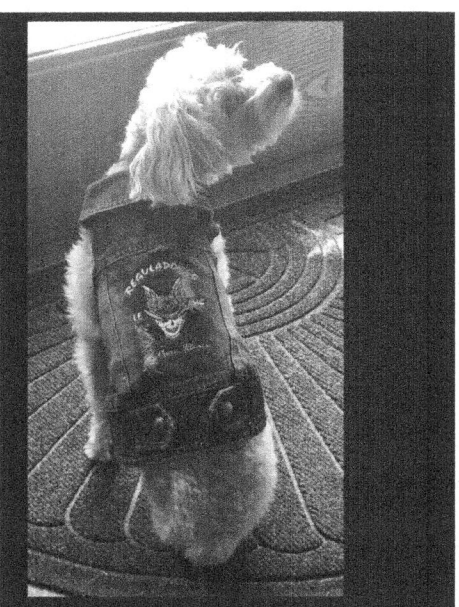

Meika rides motorcycles so she needs a "Cut". We adopted in 2017

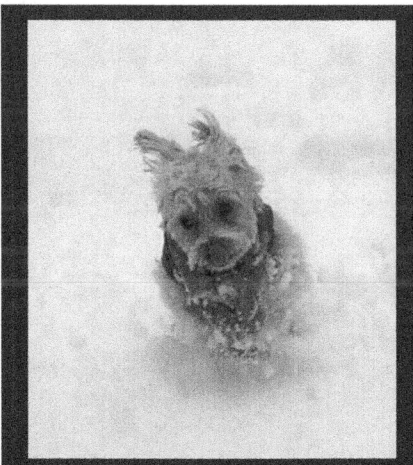

Meika our three legged deer chasing, fox playing very fast 6 lb. wonder.

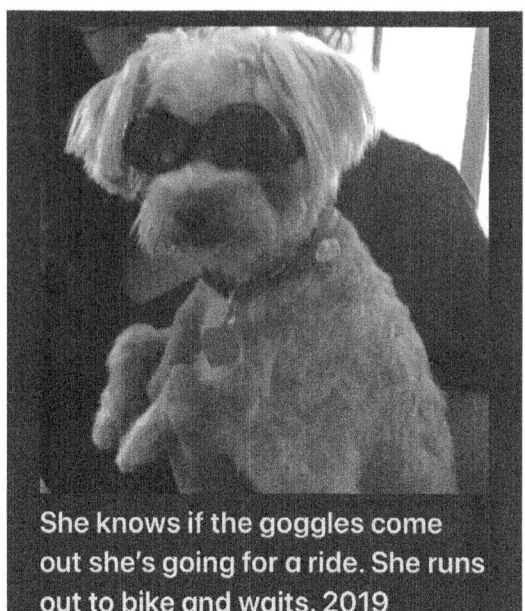

She knows if the goggles come out she's going for a ride. She runs out to bike and waits. 2019

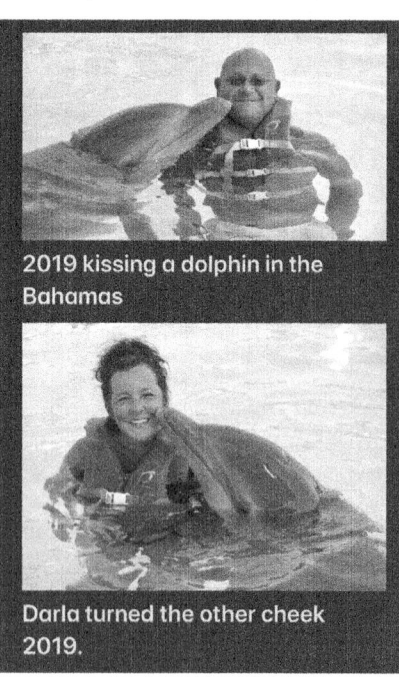

2019 kissing a dolphin in the Bahamas

Darla turned the other cheek 2019.

Sherif Gabr
Very nice pearl Dr. **Denzel D. Jines!**
You can't put this stuff in a text book chapter. This is the squeeze of a long experienced career delivered by a wise practitioner.
Good to see you again.
PS: I've never met you and you do not know me, but you've influenced my life in a very positive way by way of your past posts.
The internet can be a magical thing.
Have a nice Sunday!

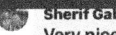 Greg Charles and 3 others

Rafi Isaac
Would love for Dr. **Denzel D. Jines** to give more insights in this format, this is great stuff!

The reason I post in Dental Clinical Pearls.

 Denzel D. Jines Differentials can include not in any specific order : needle tract infection, hematoma, joint displacement secondary to over opening or direct injection into joint space, neuropathy secondary diabetes that's poorly controlled from inadequate dietary restriction or improper medication usage or previous stated infection that necessitates altering her meds, direct trauma from the injection causing post op intramuscular edema and even eschemia(decreased vascular activity) in joint capsule(rare zebra). I will assume your patient's A1C is good(7 or less) and her diabetes is well controlled. I'll assume she had no TMJ issues prior or no medical contra indications to treatment. I would rule out infection clinically...afebrile, no adenopathy and no dysphasia, no direct edema and erythema at injection site. You can have a CBC run to check further but let's stick to clinical first.
She can swell post operatively a couple days after your procedures so if her occlusion was not altered immediately after procedure then you can safely assume this is post op phenomenon and statistically will pass within two weeks. Steroids can help alleviate symptoms;however, I am loathe to prescribe these if I can get resolution without the aggravated issues of increasing her likelihood of uncontrolled diabetes, further weakening of her immune system and increasing her chances of osteoporosis which are all consequences of lifelong accumulated steroid use. (Personally I have only seen or used steroids to actually cure just one condition...piriformis muscle syndrome everywhere absolutely everywhere else it has been perfume on body odor and nothing more). I do use short courses of steroids but again as a last resort.

Giving an answer to an emergent clinical question 2019. Staying involved.

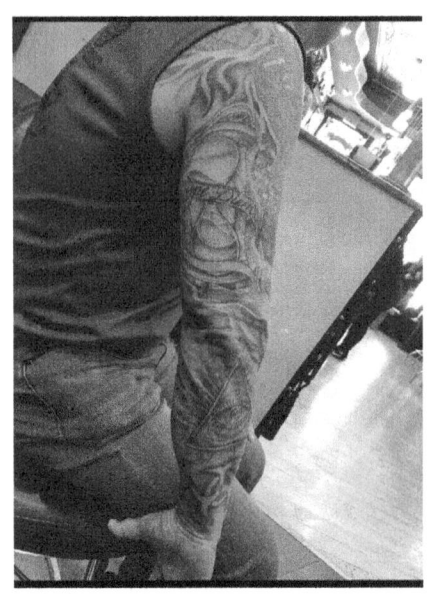

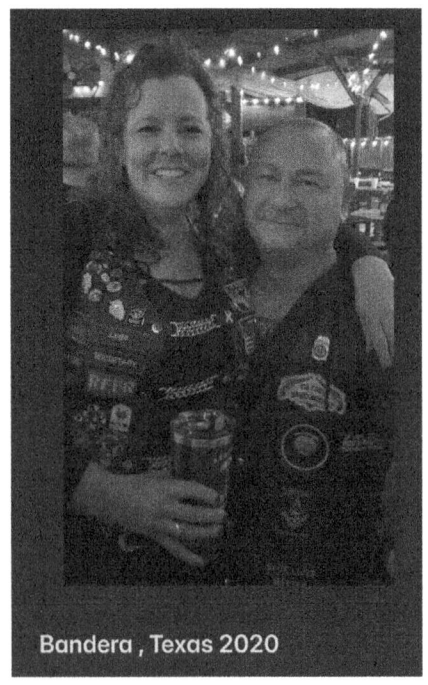

Bandera , Texas 2020

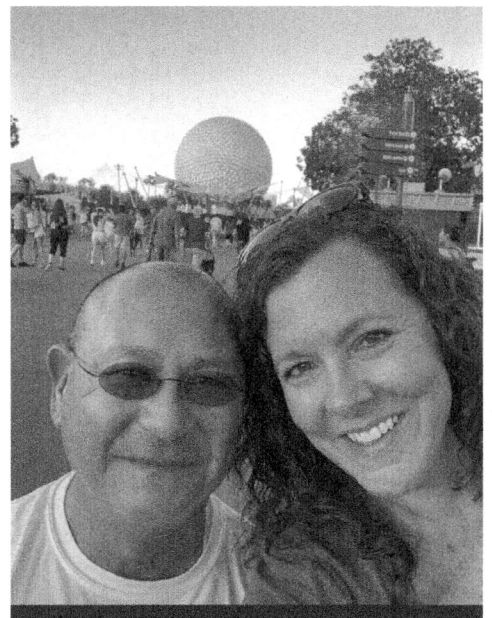

Disney 2020.

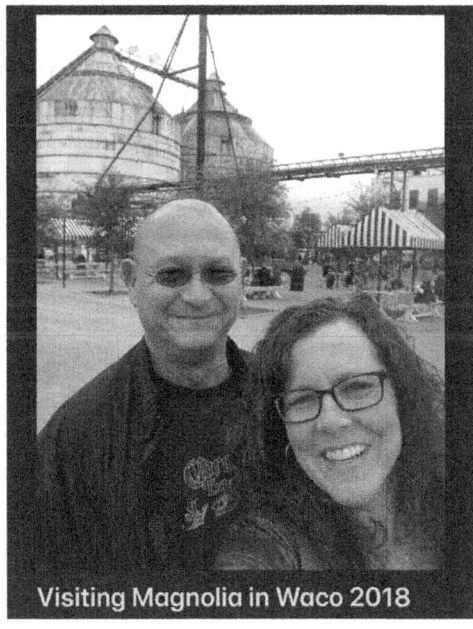

Visiting Magnolia in Waco 2018

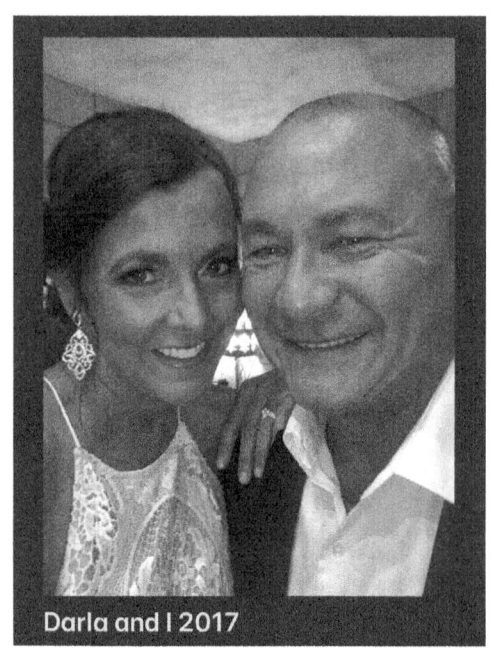

Darla and I 2017

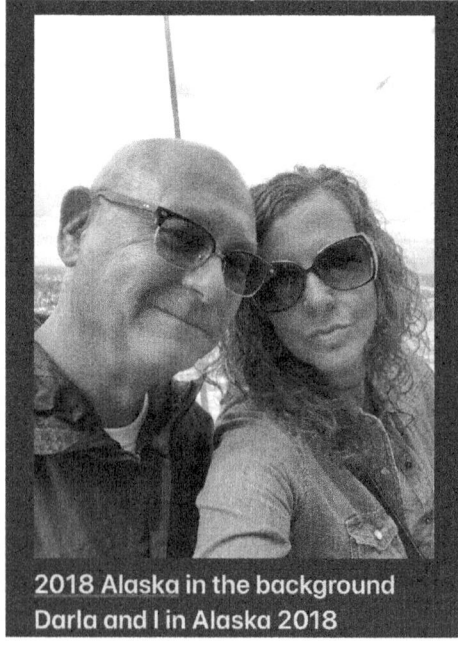

2018 Alaska in the background
Darla and I in Alaska 2018

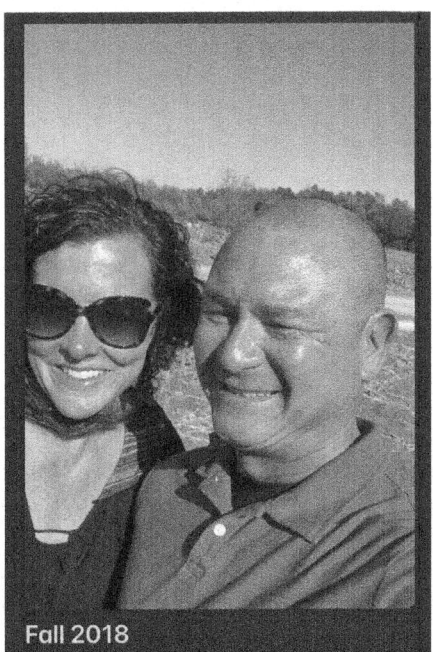

Fall 2018

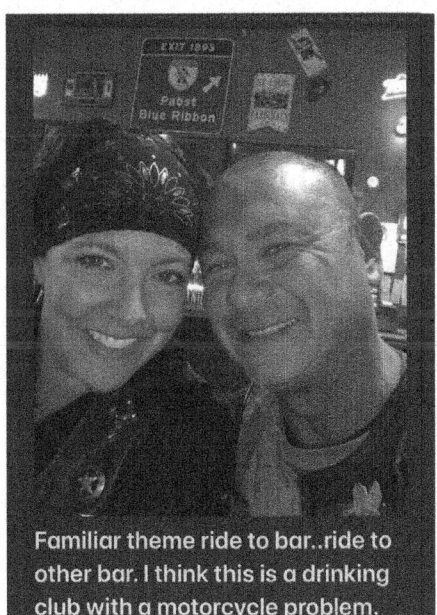

Familiar theme ride to bar..ride to other bar. I think this is a drinking club with a motorcycle problem.

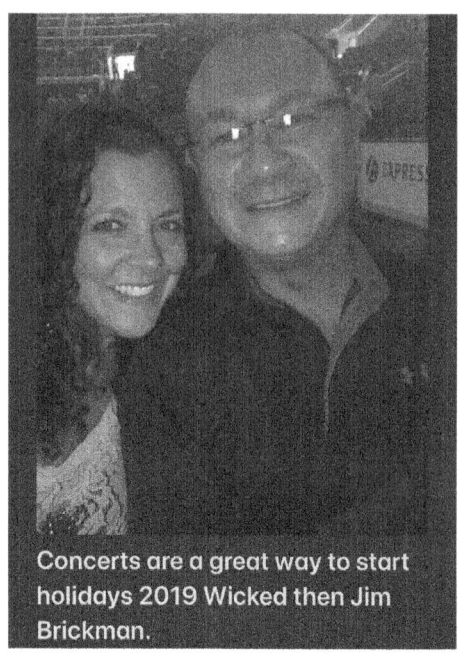

Concerts are a great way to start holidays 2019 Wicked then Jim Brickman.

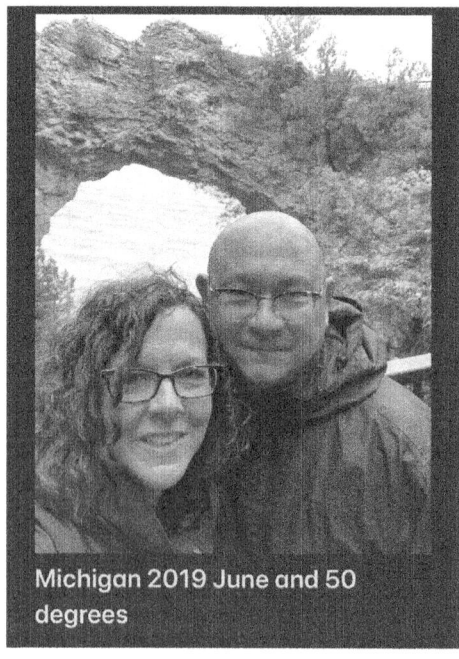

Michigan 2019 June and 50 degrees

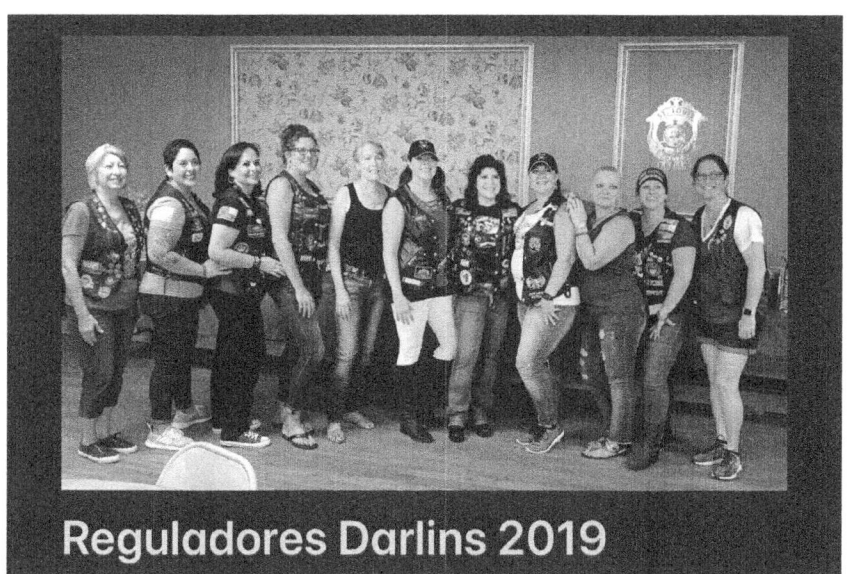

Reguladores Darlins 2019

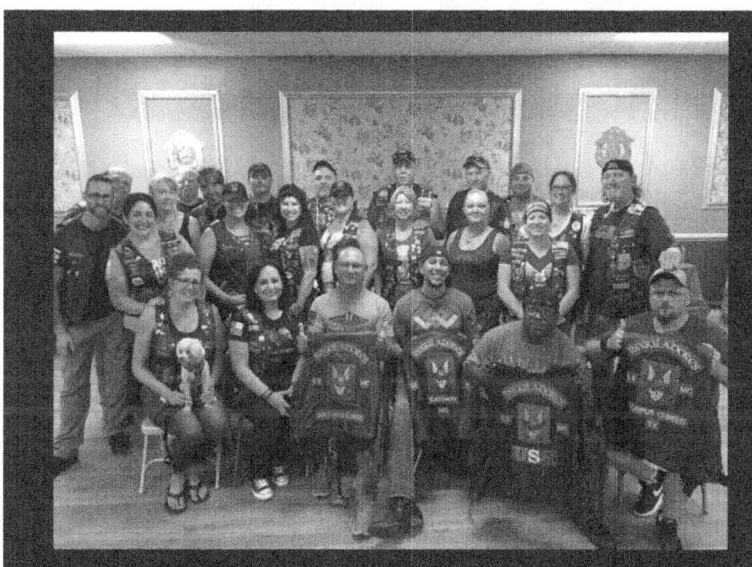

Reguladores at St. Louis Police
fund raiser. 2019

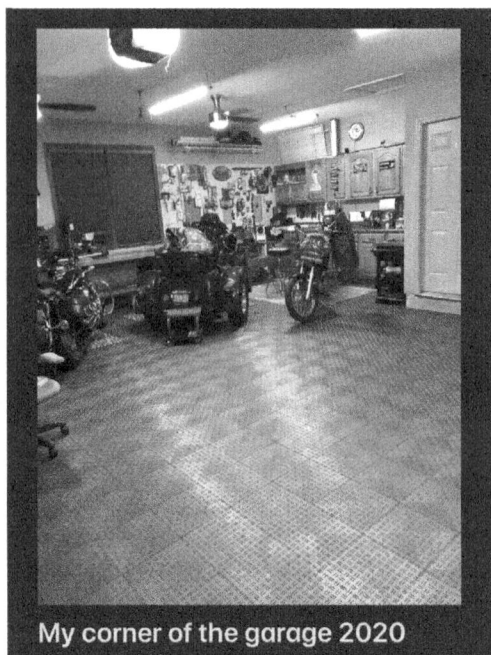

My corner of the garage 2020

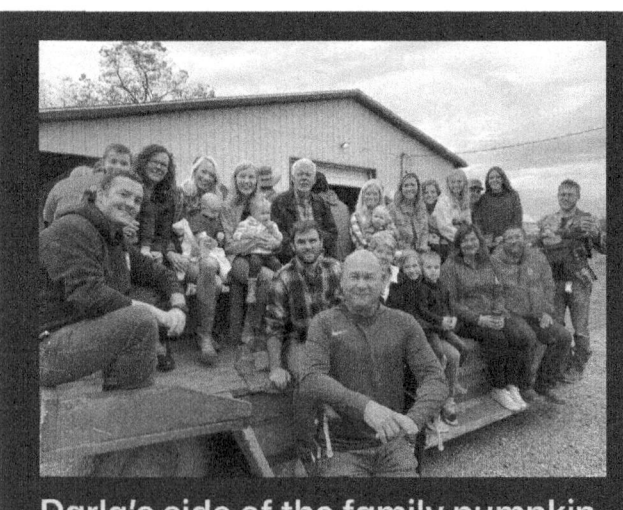

Darla's side of the family pumpkin picking 2019

2019 Christmas Party.

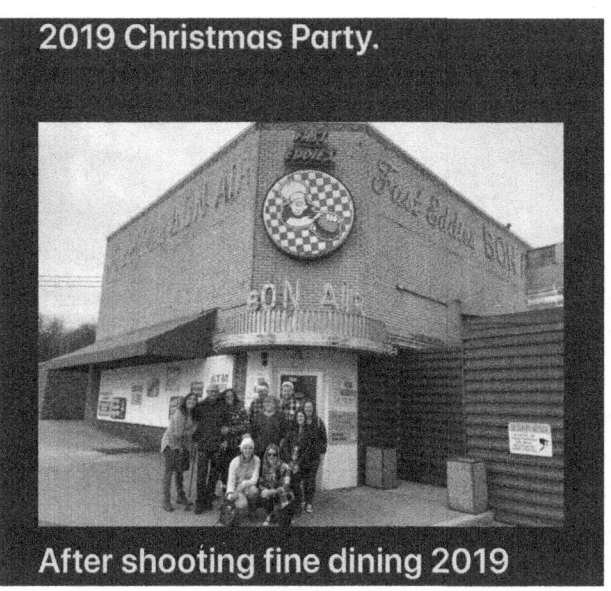

After shooting fine dining 2019

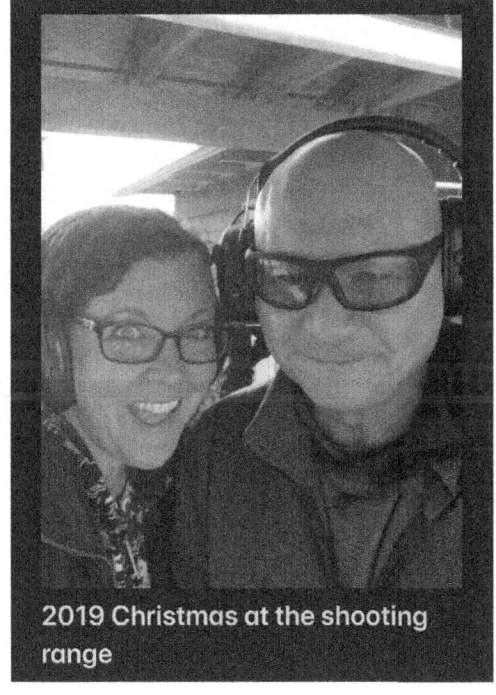

2019 Christmas at the shooting range

2019 Christmas at the shooting range

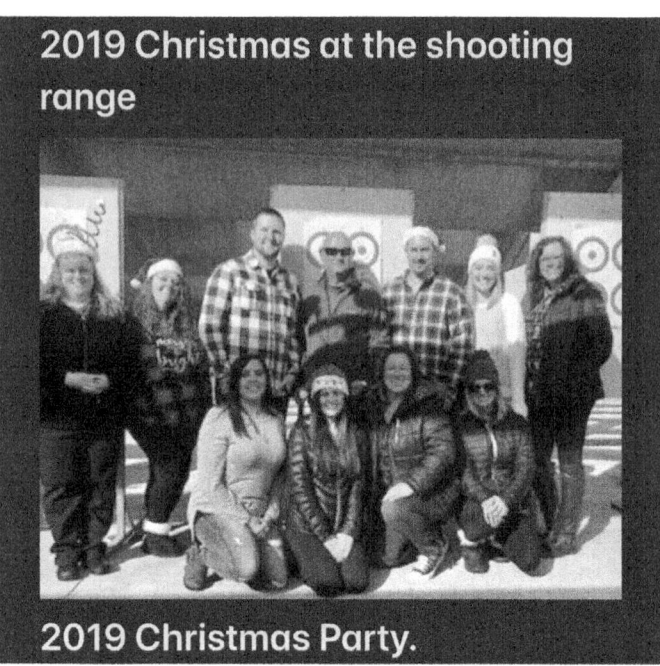

2019 Christmas Party.

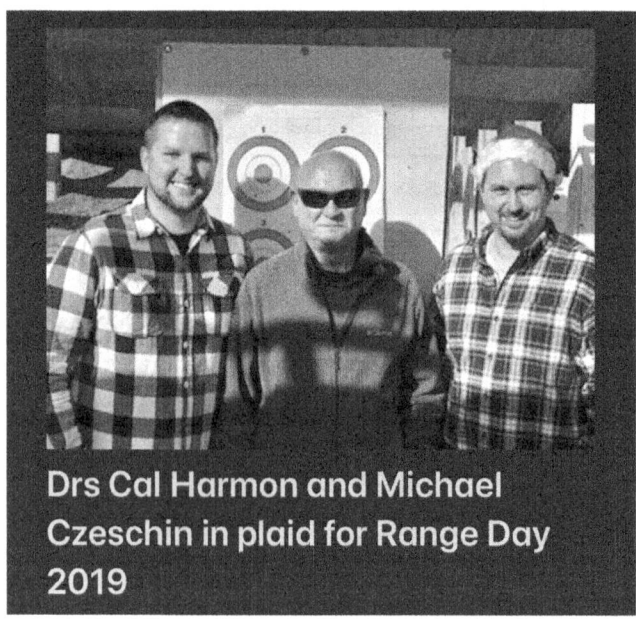

Drs Cal Harmon and Michael Czeschin in plaid for Range Day 2019

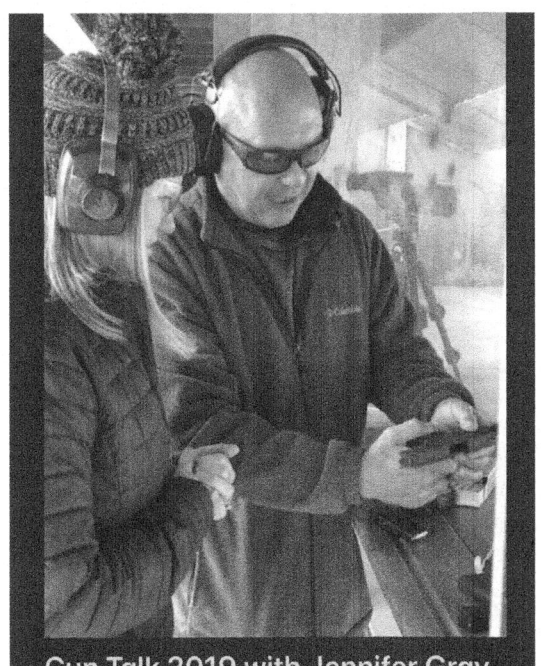

Gun Talk 2019 with Jennifer Gray

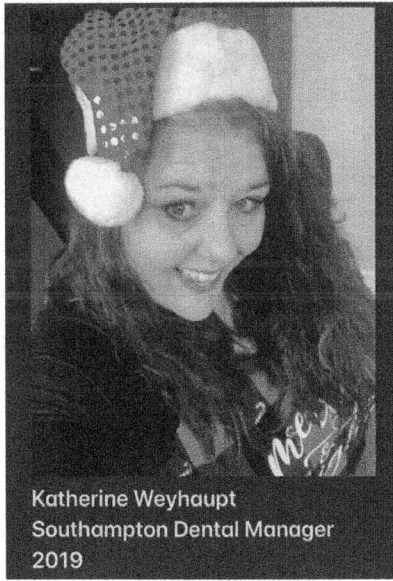

Katherine Weyhaupt
Southampton Dental Manager
2019

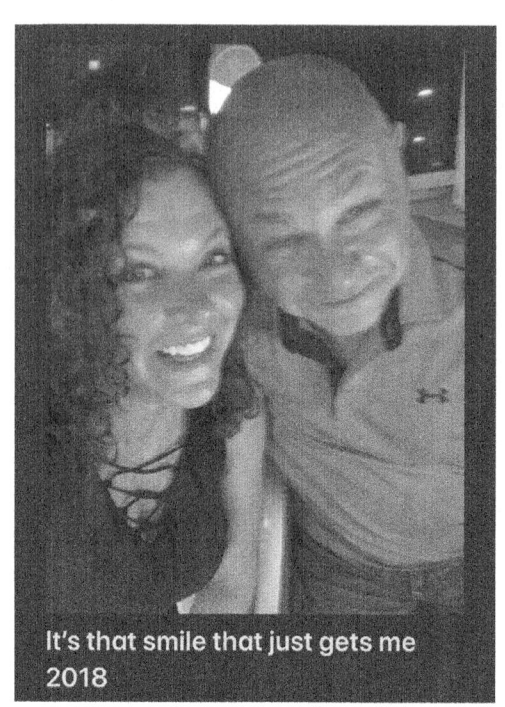

It's that smile that just gets me
2018

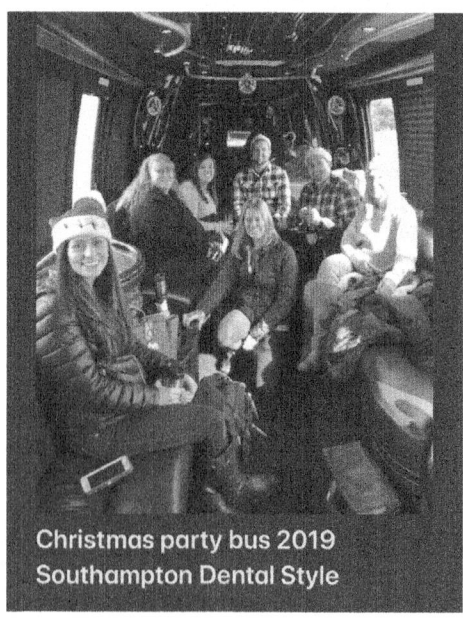

Christmas party bus 2019
Southampton Dental Style

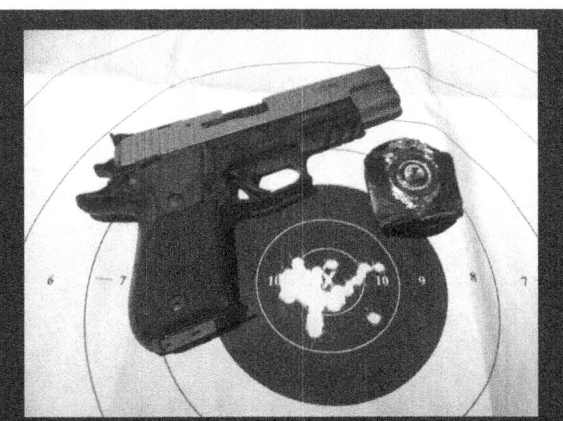

This is what 30 rounds of 45 ACP and a perfect 300 point score fired at 25 yards looks like. The Sig 220 was a graduation gift from medical school from West Point Graduate former Green Beret and friend Dr. Charles Letcher.

ACKNOWLEDGMENTS

Thanking Staff
Dr. Cal Harmon, Dr. Michael Czeschin, Katherine Weyhaupt Manager, Jennifer Gray RDH, Julie Chilton, Dawn Heidbrink RN,RDH, Kara Garrott RDH, Tracy Brust CDA, Kaleigh Love RDH, Kelley Eldridge,Tina Cracchiolo CDA

I want to thank each of you for the wonderful gifts this year. I will enjoy them. They are awesome. You all are the greatest gift I could ever have wished for. Your hard work and devotion plus your unsurpassed generosity and sacrifices made daily to our cause of fighting disease and saving lives contribute immeasurably to our community. You all surpass any measure one can take when it comes to work ethic and endurance while dealing with individuals in our very public work. I am so proud of what was created and what is being sustained through all your efforts. I love each and every one of you. My heart is full of gratitude and respect for each of you. Your individual contribution to this practice, my own personal life, and our continued friendship is what gets me in the feels whenever I am down. You all make living this life worthwhile. Peace.

Thank you to the ALS Foundation for being the essential resource we need in fighting this disease.

Thank you to the entire VA healthcare system for your support and excellent care.

Thank you Dr. David Prelutsky you have been a leader and mentor whose dedication to the LGBTQ community has saved lives as a pioneer here in the Midwest in HIV/AIDS care. You've pioneered the specialty and been instrumental in my continued training as well as my personal physician. To all my patients and friends and family a million times over.

Prayer Warriors
Thanks, Steve And Jenny

Thank you to all my prayer warriors, family, and friends, for keeping me in your thoughts. I received this special prayer request and offering from Steve and Jenny Ridings. I am humbled beyond words, and my heart is lightened constantly by you all. As Val Kilmer said to Kurt Russell at the tree after dispatching Michael Beine in the movie *Tombstone,* "Oh, I'm not as sick as I let on." I'm just me with a little baggage that I'm allowing God to carry. I highly recommend letting God take over. It is easier than you would expect, and life gets easier when you are not carrying the world's weight on your shoulders.

ABOUT THE AUTHOR

Denzel D. Jines, II, DMD, MD is a retired dentist at Southampton Dental from St. Louis, Missouri and a retired police officer. He is graduate of Washington University School of Dental Medicine, American International School of Medicine and the University of Virginia. He served the citizens of Lebanon and East Carondelet, Illinois as an officer from 1993-2016. He is a former United States Naval officer having served onboard USS Theodore Roosevelt CVN-71. While in the navy he certified as a SCUBA diver and is a private pilot. He's married to Darla and together they have 5 children and 10 grandchildren. He is the author of Appointment With Karma a novel and Before I Can't, Before I'm Gone, My ALS Story which are his Random Thoughts about his experiences dealing with ALS. Since retiring he has written two books using one thumb entirely on his iPhone.

Made in the USA
Monee, IL
15 June 2020